the love guide
Sex Talk and the Irish

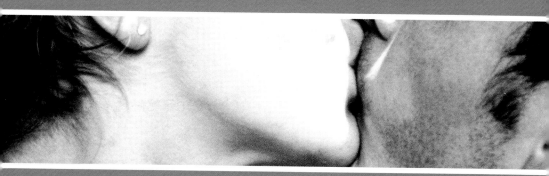

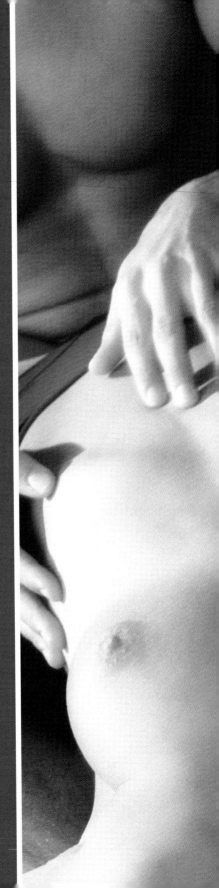

This first edition published in 2005 by
Merlin Publishing
16 Upper Pembroke Street
Dublin 2, Ireland
Tel: +353 1 676 4373
Fax: +353 1 676 4368
publishing@merlin.ie
www.merlinwolfhound.com

ISBN 1-903582-60-1

A CIP catalogue record for this book is available from
the British Library.

10 9 8 7 6 5 4 3 2 1

Cover and Internal Design by Graham Thew Design
Printed and bound by Printer Portuguesa

The Love guide

SEX TALK & THE IRISH

DR ANGELA BROKMANN

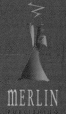

MERLIN
PUBLISHING

Acknowledgements

I wish to express my gratitude and thanks to everybody who has helped to plan and complete this book. My special thanks to Colm MacGinty and John Sheils from The Sunday World for their support.

Thanks to Aoife Barrett and Chenile Keogh from Merlin Publishing for their patience and hard work.

A sincere thanks to my survey teams, who gathered the data required. It was a tough task, and you did a great job.

And many thanks to everybody who has openly shared their most intimate thoughts and experiences which appear as real life quotes throughout the book.

Contents

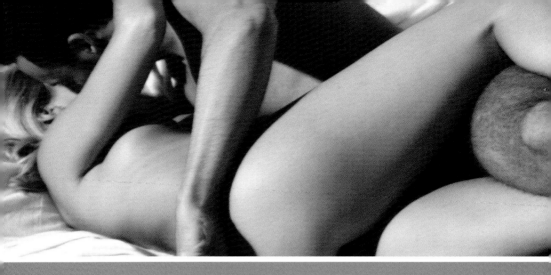

Introduction

How's your sex life? Are you purring with satisfaction or just getting by? Are you happy or do you feel that there might be something else out there – to catapult you into higher spheres of pleasure?

No matter how happy or full of desire you are *The Love Guide* will answer your questions and change your love life for the better. It is not only based on my more than 20 years experience as a sexologist and sex therapist, it also encapsulates the results of a survey I conducted with almost 600 Irish men and women, who were asked about the most intimate details of their sex lives. The survey was nation-wide, covering ages ranging from 16 to 40, and the results prove very interesting!

Finding the right person can be hard and it usually starts with flirting. Flirting is much more than winking an eye or delivering a cheeky chat-up line. Flirting is an art, which needs to be mastered to guarantee success. You don't have to be a natural sex bomb you just need to find out how to send the right messages and how to interpret signals so that you capture and allure your prey. Having sex appeal makes life easier and with the tips and tricks in The Love Guide everybody can increase their chances of being sexy and desirable.

Once you've found a lover it can be even tougher to keep them satisfied. Erotic love means much more than mere enjoyment and ecstasy. It is about giving and receiving pleasure. This guide highlights many of the best ways to make love to each other. Find out the different ways that men and women enjoy being caressed and how to improve your bedroom antics. For example most people know by now that it's harder for women to climax during intercourse than it is for men. We will look at how women can best achieve an orgasm and discuss what can be done during foreplay to ensure that HER level of arousal at least matches HIS. Learn the best ways to get yourself and your partner into the right mood, how to let your hands and lips glide all over your lover's body to tantalise them and how to kiss their body from top to toe, teasing their most sensitive spots – the erogenous zones.

The opposite sex is often a mystery, which can attract and dismay us at the same time. This book unveils many of the mysteries and myths that have fuelled lovers' imagination throughout the ages. Get inspired by the Kama Sutra, the ancient art of love. Find out if men constantly think of sex. Are women really more demure? Is there such a thing as love at first sight? Are Irish men good lovers and what about Irish women?

When it comes to the choice of sex positions male and female preferences often clash. While most women love the missionary position, Irish men, for example, prefer their women to be on top and in charge. The survey also revealed that, on average, Irish people only know 12 different ways to make love. So we'll look at the favourite sex positions, as well as checking out many new exotic ones.

Playing erotic games is another great way to spice up your love life. Making love under water is the most popular sex game in Ireland. You can enjoy this in the sea, in a hot tub, or even in the shower. The Love Guide also explores other ways to make your love life more exciting, including erotic massage, exhibitionism, fetishism, and the lustful pains of BDSM.

In a loving relationship, you should realise that your partner's sexual needs and wishes are just as important as your own. Communication is crucial for improving sexual satisfaction and maintaining each partner's confidence in the relationship, so open up, and talk about your dreams and desires. Ask yourself how much you know about your partner's wishes and fantasies and how much does your partner know about yours? There are lots of sexual fantasies that people keep a secret. Don't expect your partner to have a sixth sense that decodes the vibes you are sending out. You need to give them, at least some, clues about your preferences.

In general, in my many years working in this sphere, I have discovered that if you have a playful and creative attitude towards sex you'll have more fun. Since having sex and a loving relationship not only makes us happy, but also dramatically improves our mental and physical health, there are many good reasons to strive for a fulfilling love life – even doctors recommend it!

Dr Angela Brokmann
2005

Erogenous Zones

The erogenous zones are the most sensitive parts of our body – the hot spots of desires. These zones, when touched, kissed and teased make your skin tingle and your heart beat faster.

The genitals are about the only erogenous zone we all have in common. Beyond that there are huge differences between men and women, with personal tastes complicating the matter even more. Both male and female genitals are packed with highly sensory nerve endings that almost inevitably respond with sexual arousal when triggered.

It is a widespread prejudice that men have basically only one erogenous zone – their genitals – while women have many mysterious zones of pleasure, widely spread all over their body. As with many prejudices, there is a hint of truth in this one. Most guys are happy enough when you go for their genitals straightaway, while women normally expect you to concentrate on less obvious erogenous parts of their anatomy first, like the back of their thighs.

Men have those mystery spots as well, although they might not be aware of it. There are plenty more erogenous zones on their bodies that are worth exploring. It is very rewarding to find an erotic sensitive area on your lover's body that he didn't even know about.

So where are these hot spots that will drive your lover mad with desire? It's impossible to draw a general map of our erogenous zones but we can highlight where men and women are most sensitive and examine how they love to be caressed in those areas. The following serves as a guideline to find your partner's most sensitive spots. Take your time to playfully explore each other's bodies. Keep in mind that your partner probably doesn't know all their personal hot spots. There should still be some unexplored areas of pleasure. It's up to you to find them.

Erogenous Zones

Irish Women's TOP 7 Sensitive Spots

Genitals	85%
Breasts	62%
Nape of the neck	51%
Buttocks	46%
Back	42%
Lips	37%
Scalp	35%

Irish Men's TOP 7 Sensitive Spots

Genitals	94%
Inner thighs	54%
Loins	46%
Nape of the neck	44%
Throat	43%
Lower belly	36%
Lips	34%

Women's TOP 7 Erogenous Zones

Genitals It is no surprise that women love their clitoris being stimulated. But to arouse a woman that way or even make her orgasm is not a simple task. It doesn't happen by just pressing the right button. You need to get your touch right, to apply the exact amount of pressure at the right time and on the correct spot.

The clitoris and surrounding area can be stimulated either by hand, by lips or by tongue. Most women prefer circulating movements of either fingers or tongue around the clitoris, starting slowly and gently, and then proceeding with increasing speed and pressure. Get it right, and you'll be rewarded with little moans and gasps. If your lover starts to squirm, make sure it's out of pleasure and not discomfort. The difference isn't hard to tell: when a woman gets sexually aroused, her vagina starts secreting fluids to prepare for inter-course. By gently slipping a fingertip in, you can easily check the progress of your efforts. Gently move your finger inside her while you keep caressing her clitoris for additional stimulation. But be careful: not all women like being 'fingered'. Pull back if she shows any signs of displeasure.

Breasts Men don't need a special invitation to touch and caress a woman's breasts. Not because they know that a woman's breasts – especially her nipples – are highly sensitive, but primarily for their own pleasure. Breasts just have a magic force of attraction and are highly sensitive at the same time. The more sensitive they are, the more difficult they are to handle.

Almost all Irish women, (89%), like their breasts being softly caressed. After that, the tastes vary: every second woman loves to have her breasts kissed and licked, especially the soft area below the nipples and the outer sides near her armpits. Feeling their lover responding, most guys go for more than gentle caresses and therefore invite disaster. They fulfil their desire to suck her nipples, which only one out of every six women appreciates.

So there you are again, facing the old dilemma – you will never find out what makes your partner horny without trying. So don't take little setbacks to heart, don't be put off by rejection. The best you can do is to explore what turns her on gently and patiently. After all, some women fancy much more than just caressing, so it's worth trying out sexy games as well as the every day techniques. Here's a few hints which might be worth a try: one out of every ten women likes to get her nipples pinched and as many love gentle love bites. And one out of five women loves to feel her partner's erect penis rubbing against her breasts. As a special kick, let the tip of your penis tease her nipple. Also worth a try: be playfully rough and gently slap your erect penis against her breasts.

'My current lover was the first to touch my breasts with his penis,' confesses Caroline (23) from Co. Cavan. 'He first teases me by letting his penis tip circle around my nipple. He then puts the very tip of his penis above my nipple, taking it in, pretending I'm making love to him with my erect nipple. It is the most amazing feeling, especially if he comes this way.'

3 Nape of the Neck

Stroking, kissing, and nibbling your lover's nape of her neck will most surely make her quiver with pleasure. Gently massage her neck, and then follow your hands with your mouth. Let your teeth and lips nibble on her neck, while you move your massaging hands into her hairline. If you want to spoil your lover without expecting much for yourself, take the nape of her neck as the starting point for a relaxing and arousing back massage.

4 Buttocks

One out of two women likes the feeling of her lover's hands and lips on her bottom. Richly supplied with sensory nerve endings, the buttocks are perfect spots for gentle fondling, squeezing and kneading. Erotic kisses and gentle love bites are appreciated as well. Let your lips and tongue glide over the bum's smooth skin. Use your teeth to softly nibble on her flesh. If that gives her goosebumps of pleasure all over, try a very gentle, playful bite. Gently nibble and suck while you hold her flesh with your teeth. While your mouth is busy nibbling on her buttocks, stroke the underside of her bum and her inner thighs with your hands. Be very careful with caressing her anus. Some women like being touched there, but for most it's a real turn off, especially when your fingers get too inquisitive and try to slip in. But again – some women love it, so it's worth checking out.

As a little treat for yourself, use the tip of your penis to tease her buttocks. Gently squeeze them together to rub yourself between them. For a steamy bit of teasing, lightly sit on her bum, with your penis amusing itself with her buttocks, while your hands and mouth work on your lover's neck, back and shoulders.

5 Back

A woman's back does not have much erotic appeal from a man's point of view – the buttocks can be sexy, but often the back itself is no big turn on. Women are well aware of this, so it counts all the more if you make a real effort to spoil her by stroking, kissing and especially massaging her back. You can't go wrong with simply stroking her back all over. For a bit more finesse, follow your lover's spine with your tongue, while you gently stroke and massage the sides of her lower back. This shouldn't fail to make her shiver all over and squirm under your hands with pleasure.

For a gentle back massage, sit on her naked behind to let her feel your penis against her buttocks, then massage her shoulders and back. You will hear her moan and purr with pleasure. The only problem is it feels so good that she'll never want you to stop. To coax her around, move your penis between her upper thighs to tease her clitoris, and then it can sneakily find its way in. As long as you keep massaging, she probably won't interfere.

'My girlfriend is absolutely mad about back massage', groans Michael (34), 'but it's a real turn off for me. I even used to lose my erection while I was working on her back to please her. Now we have found a compromise that's satisfying for both of us: she gets her back massage, while I rub my penis between her buttocks and her thighs. After about 20 minutes of this, she invitingly lifts her bum up to make it easier for me to slip inside her. If she forgets, I teasingly remind her by slapping her bum with my erect penis.'

6 Lips A man has to be good at kissing to impress a woman. So if you master the art of kissing, licking and nibbling her lips you have a very good chance of turning your partner on. A good kiss will make her long for more. Start playing with her upper and bottom lip while embracing and caressing her. Trace the outside of her lips lightly with your fingertip, and then trace the inside with your tongue. Let your tongue slip in and teasingly move around hers. When your kiss gets more passionate after all this teasing, your lover will respond eagerly.

7 Scalp A woman's scalp is another one of those places that guys don't fancy attending to. Lots of women long for a bit of teasing here, so give it a try. Move your hands from her neck upwards into her hairline. Gently massage her scalp with your fingertips in small circling movements. Lightly touch and scratch behind her ears – I'm not joking! It's not only dogs that like being scratched behind their ears. For a special treat, give your lover a head massage. For a bit of erotic flair, do it in the shower or bathtub. Wash her hair and then spoil her by massaging her scalp.

Men's TOP 7 Erogenous Zones

I Genitals *A man's genitals are the top erotic zone of his body. Although they are extremely sensitive, it is not easy to please them, especially as every man has his own preferences. In the most basic caress you simply stroke and squeeze the shaft of his penis. Your partner can show you what amount of pressure he likes by putting his hand over your own while you are holding him. Vary the amount of pressure while your hand goes up and down to see what suits your man best. If you feel that you are getting it wrong, ask him to put his hand over yours and make himself come that way. Next time, you can try to copy his technique. The penis head is much more sensitive than the shaft. Tender caresses with lips and tongue are therefore much more appreciated than a rubbing hand. However to expertly stimulate the tip of his penis by hand, touch it gently but make sure your hands are slippery with lubricant before you start.*

A man's testicles are even more sensitive. They can be extremely ticklish; so it is better not to tease them with too light a touch. On the other hand, make sure you don't squeeze them too heartily, for anything above a very gentle squeeze is prone to hurt badly. As a special treat, kiss and lick his testicles while your hands are caressing his penis. Even better, do it the other way around: kiss his penis, while your hands hold and caress his testicles.

'I often make my man come just by teasing his penis with my hands. He likes it best when I rub my hands with massage oil before I enclose his penis with my fist', describes Helen (23) from Co. Waterford. 'First I only cup the head of his penis with my hand, holding him firmly with my fist closed on top, not letting him slip out that way. After a couple of minutes, I let him squeeze through, and rub his shaft for a while. Then I enclose his tip again. It almost drives him mad with desire. He struggles to break through my grip again, and when I finally let him he orgasms.'

2 Inner Thighs *Before you go for a man's penis or testicles, caress the tender area of his inner thighs. Being highly sensitive, without being overly ticklish, a man's inner thighs are the perfect spot for teasing. Keep your touch* light. The more accidental your caresses seem to be, the more exciting they are. When you feel that your touch is exciting your partner, let your fingertips glide slightly over his perineum and then finally brush lightly against his scrotum. The perineum is the area between testicles and anus. This won't fail to make him yearn for more. For the ultimate turn on, move your lips slightly over the skin of your man's inner thighs. Let your mouth glide slowly but steadily towards his scrotum in a tantalising promise for even more intense pleasure.

3 Loins *Your man's loins are another ideal part of his body to play with. Being very close to his genitals, caressing of this highly sensitive area almost involuntarily brings about an erection. Just a few fleeting touches – and pop, up he goes. Men love to have their loins kissed. To drive him mad with desire, caress and kiss his loins at length. Let your hands and lips move slowly towards his genitals. Almost there, draw back teasingly and then start to move in again. Brush your mouth against his genitals fleetingly, as if by mistake, and then pull back again. Keep going until he surrenders and begs for more.*

4 Nape of the Neck *The nape of a man's neck is the perfect place for passionate kisses and tender massages. Gently massage him with your fingertips in circling movements, and then let your*

hands move into his hairline. The nape of his neck shouldn't be as ticklish as his throat, so you can kiss him there without giving him the giggles. Try nibbling and gentle biting as well, while you let one of your hands play with his hairline.

5 Throat *The throat is a very sensual spot of the male body that is not located in the immediate vicinity of the genitals for a change. Nevertheless, your man's throat is an incredible erotic zone that invites kissing, licking, sucking and gentle nibbling. Move your lips and tongue over the area under his jawbone. If he's not ticklish, try soft sucking, just be careful not to leave marks. When guys have their very first girlfriend they might wear love bites proudly as proof of their success with the girls. But growing out of their teens, most guys find it most inconvenient to have to cover their love marks when they go to work the next morning.*

6 Lower Belly *For a special and tantalising treat, have a go at your man's lower belly; it's an ideal playground for teasing. Stroke and kiss his belly below the belly button, moving slowly but surely towards the root of his penis. Let the back of your fingers glide over both sides of his belly, while your mouth nibbles in the middle. You will be rewarded by his penis stretching out to meet your lips while you keep* touching and kissing the tender skin of his belly. Don't go for his genitals yet, only brush your mouth and hands fleetingly against them for another while. Finally, you will have to show mercy and pay some attention to his penis as well.

'My girl's teasing is like a tantalising pleasurable torture,' describes Denis (28). 'My lower belly is my second favourite spot for caressing. My girlfriend takes shameless advantage of that. She caresses me lightly, almost tickling for minutes on end, moving ever closer to my penis, but avoiding touching it. The ultimate torture is when she lifts my penis up from my belly, holding it uncaringly between thumb and forefinger, while she strokes the area underneath it.'

7 Lips One out of three guys counts his lips as one of his most erogenous zones. To see whether your man is one of them, take the lead. Hold his head, trace his bottom lip with a fingertip, and tell him in your husky voice that you would love to kiss him. Move his face closer, but don't kiss him yet, put him on tenterhooks. Describe how you would love to kiss him. Start nibbling on his lips while you tell him. He will melt under your hands and lips.

SEX DICTIONARY

EROGENOUS ZONES

Erogenous zones are areas of the body that are especially sensitive to sexual stimulation. Touching or kissing these areas leads to sexual arousal.

GENITALS

Medical term for external and internal male and female reproductive organs. Often used as generic term for mainly external organs involved in sex: the male penis and testicles, and the female clitoris, labia and vagina.

PERINEUM

Highly sensitive, but much neglected area between genitals and anus.

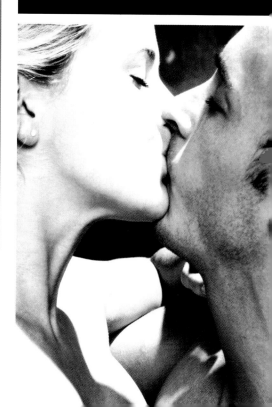

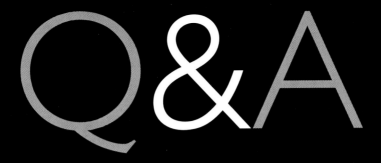

Q&A

I caress my man in all the spots that I am sensitive in, but I can tell that he doesn't like it – what's wrong?

Tease HIS hot spots, not the ones YOU fancy. You can't take it for granted that your lover is most sensitive in the same areas as yourself. More likely than not, his hot zones are completely different from yours. To please your man, explore his body to find out where he likes to be stroked, kissed and teased.

How can an inexperienced guy like me find his girlfriend's clitoris without too much fumbling and making a fool of himself?

The clitoris is located at the tip of the vaginal entrance. To find it, place your hand on your girlfriend's lower belly and from there move it down through her pubic hair towards the area between her thighs, with your fingertips pointing downwards. Move slowly until you feel a tiny knob that sticks out under your fingertips – that's the clitoris. If you don't manage to find it at first just move your fingertips slowly up and then down again. To distract your girlfriend's attention from your mission, give her a steamy kiss at the same time.

How should I caress and kiss his testicles? He gets squeamish every time I try.

A man's testicles are very sensitive and vulnerable but don't let that spoil your fun, just treat them tenderly. Weigh your man's testicles in the palm of your hand, holding them in a very loose grip without pressing or squeezing. When you make oral love, let your tongue and lips glide over them. You need to be very careful with sucking, and should avoid biting games altogether, unless your man encourages it.

Since I gave birth, I love my man to nibble my nipples and suck my breasts. I feel bad about having those sexual feelings when my breasts should be reserved for my baby.

There is no harm in what you are doing, and definitely no need to feel bad about it. You are not the only couple enjoying this love game, many others do the same. Often men lust after their women's breasts even more when they swell with pregnancy and childbirth. Women have mixed feelings about this. Some feel too sensitive and sore to wish for any love games that include their breasts, others are reluctant to give in to erotic longings, being too focused on their babies. But more and more young mothers enjoy the increased sensitivity of their breasts during pregnancy and after childbirth, and simply enjoy these special erotic feelings.

We love to fondle and kiss each other's feet – Are we perverts?

All areas of the body are potential erogenous zones, whether it's your feet, your scalp or anything in between. There are a few hot spots like the penis and clitoris that enjoy widespread popularity, while other areas like arms or feet are more exclusive. The fact that there are not many others who share your desire does not mean you are a pervert. You just have a different taste and there is nothing wrong with that.

My partner never cuddles and teases me before we make love. He just goes for my clitoris straight away. Are all guys like that or am I just unlucky?

Not all men are the same, most spend some time cuddling before they go for more – not necessarily because they like it, but because they know that women expect them to. The problem is that lots of men wouldn't mind a woman going for their genitals more or less straight away, without 'wasting' time on less arousing bits. So if they get away with it, they treat their women like they would like to be treated themselves, and go straight for her hottest goodies. To put a stop to this and get the attention and tenderness you need, you have to tell your man that you want to cuddle and tease. Teach him where you would like to be touched. Don't let him get away with excuses like he doesn't know about such stuff or that he is too clumsy.

2 Erotic Attraction

Erotic attraction is one of life's greatest mysteries. What are the forces that draw us towards each other? Is it a question of fate? Is it animal magnetism, chemistry, or plain old love at first sight? Are we born either with sex appeal or without it? Why is it that some folks are mad about you and think you're irresistible, while others don't even notice you?

Sexual allurement depends on mutual attraction. You might make one guy or girl melt on the spot, while another won't bother to give you a second glance, although you're sending out exactly the same signals each time. To unveil some of the mysteries of eroctic attraction, let's have a look at the factors that, often unconsciously, rule our sexual response to others.

Sexual attraction is mainly based on first appearance. You meet somebody and it just clicks. You feel an unmistakable warm sensation, a stirring in your loins or, for people who insist on being romantic, a flutter in your heart. If it doesn't hit you quite that hard, you should still feel an irresistible pull that you'd find hard to explain or to even understand yourself.

'I once met this bloke at a party,' explains Susan (23) from Dublin. 'First I could see only his back with those broad shoulders from afar, but the way he just stood there made me want to move closer. Getting close enough to hear his voice I felt shivers rippling down my spine, although I still hadn't even seen his face. When I stood behind him, he turned around, as though he had sensed me standing there. He looked into my eyes, gave me a gorgeous smile and we started chatting away as though we had known each other for ages. It didn't take us long to leave the party, we just couldn't keep our hands off each other. It was only a one-night stand in the end, but a fabulous one!'

The Three Senses

When we notice a prospective partner three of our senses are involved, more or less on impact: sight, sound and smell. We can instantly tell from his or her looks whether we find a person attractive. We hear somebody talk or laugh, or just shuffle around, and feel excited, neutral or put off. Then – believe it or not! – our sense of smell comes into play. Your nose may react to a scent and find it arousing, exciting, agreeable, boring or disgusting. And there are mysterious hormonal smells involved in attraction that we are not even consciously aware of.

So let's have a closer look at how these three senses effect your erotic attractiveness.

Sight

You don't have to look gorgeous to be sexually attractive but it helps. Having the traditional hour-glass figure – ample bosom, narrow waist and voluptuous hips – is still the biggest advantage. Men with broad shoulders are in luck as well, as most women still find this type of physique attractive. Even if you aren't turned on by bodybuilders or girls who are more than skin and bones the old natural biological pull still works like an undercurrent, pulling you in the right direction, sometimes even against your personal preferences, whispering 'those shoulders will protect you' or 'she's the one to bear your children.'

Of course, physique isn't the only criteria involved when we judge our potential mates. Your general appearance, charisma and body language are also scrutinised by possible partners. If you look healthy and fit, stylish and appear confident and funny, you are on the right track.

Don't scream in protest, we are talking about biology here and although humankind is evolving, the pulls of nature still have an unconscious hold on all of us. In many ways of course civilisation is taking over, making our tastes swing more and more from the biological ideal to current cultural preferences. This also effects our own personal preferences, which become intertwined with the cultural ones. The huge impact of our personal preferences often gives suitors the chance to compensate for any underlying biological ideals that they might not shape up to. Once they have passed the visual test, they can move on to the second stage which is all about sounding good.

Sound

Your sexual attractiveness also depends on the way you sound – your manner of speaking, the language you use, the way you laugh and much more. Even the click of your heels can decide your fate. Or the way you tap your fingernails or noisily scratch your scalp when you get nervous.

The most attractive voice sounds calm and confident, with a husky undertone in intimate encounters. Loud booming voices can be a real turnoff. Don't raise your voice or interrupt people. Avoid foul language – you might find it cool to swear and curse, but it definitely works against you in terms of attractiveness. Sorry girls, but this especially goes for us. A real plus is if you laugh a lot but not so loud that you're turning heads.

'The worst a guy can do,' explains Elaine (27) from Co. Dublin, 'is to shout all over the place to draw attention. He might turn a few heads, but it doesn't make him sexy.'

'The same goes for women,' counters John (31) from Co. Donegal. 'It's nice to hear a soft giggle or a chuckling laugh, but when it gets too loud and intense, it only sounds hysterical, not sexy at all.'

Try to avoid making annoying noises, like clicking your fingernails, tapping your feet or wobbling your chair. All they do for you is to make people nervous and uncomfortable in your presence, which completely ruins your chances in the erotic department. It's not easy to get it right, but it's not too tough to avoid the worst turn-offs, and that alone improves your rating by a couple of points.

If you pass this second stage as well then you're onto stage three and all you need to do is smell right!

Smell

The way you smell, whether it's natural or artificial, can be attractive or repulsive or anything in between. The way we smell depends on different factors: our hormones, what we eat and drink, our health, and of course hygiene and the use of various lotions and potions.

It's pretty obvious that a rancid body odour won't score you any points on the erotic scale but it also works against you if you try to erase all traces of your natural smell by dousing yourself in artificial scents. A whiff of perfume can be erotic, but if you're coated in an eye-watering cloud of the stuff, anyone with sensitive smell will stay well clear of you.

'I used to go out with this gorgeous guy,' tells Mary (32) from Co. Dublin. 'We got along great, he was fun to be with. But the smell of him completely turned me off. I don't mean his natural odour, but this body spray he was using. Every time we spent a night together, he disappeared into the bathroom before we went to bed and sprayed this stuff all over him. I love to nuzzle a man's body from head to toe, but with this guy it was like licking a bottle of aftershave.'

What you eat and drink can also be a big turn off. Not only the obvious lust killers like garlic or onions can make you smell bad, but spicy food can make you stink and the smell of alcohol can be revolting as well. Alcohol is not only on your breath, it literally pours out of your skin.

The smell emitted by our pheromones is another factor that determines our erotic attractiveness. A pheromone is a chemical that's produced by the body to transmit messages to other people's sense of smell. It is still controversial in the scientific world whether humans really use pheromones for olfactory communication or not but recent studies have shown that pheromones aren't mere fiction – they actually exist. Sex pheromones are thought to be responsible for the instant attraction people feel towards one another, especially if it's somebody the guy or girl wouldn't usually find attractive.

What if I fail the Test of the Three Senses?

Although first appearance has the biggest impact, sight, sound and smell aren't all that count. You don't have to be a beauty to be sexually attractive. It does help to have good looks, but there is no need to hang your head if you are not supermodel material; with the right charisma you more than make up for it. You can still appear sexually attractive to somebody even if you don't hit it off on the spot. You might impress with your personality or the fact that you are great fun to be with or you might share common interests. There are many factors that give you a second chance but without the advantage of instant attraction, you will have to work much harder to get noticed.

When it comes to erotic attractiveness there are a wild mix of other influences that effect how erotic a person appears. Some factors have an impact that we aren't even aware of, while others depend on our personal preferences. Let's have a look at what consciously stirs our sexual interest.

The Sex Appeal Survey

Out of hundreds of people surveyed around Ireland the results of what makes Irish men and women sexy are as follows:

Top Five– Sex Appeal

HER	
Erotic Body Language	55%
Sense of Humour	49%
Self-assuredness	45%
Sexy Outfit	44%
Irresistible Smile	41%

HIM	
Erotic Body Language	64%
Irresistible Smile	58%
Protective Instinct	49%
Fascinating Eyes	44%
Charisma	39%

What Makes A Woman Sexy?

1 Erotic Body Language *Our body language gives away more about our character and attitude than we realise. Try to avoid postures and gestures that make you look clammed up and uninterested. Don't slump your shoulders, pick your nails or tap your feet. Keep your shoulders straight to show off your chest. Move your hands languidly over your body, like you're caressing yourself. Don't feel shy as you fleetingly touch your breasts. It will drive the guys mad, and make them eager to show you how much better their own hands would feel on your body. To find out more about body language, and how you can make it work for you, have a look at my flirting tips on page 33.*

2 Sense of Humour *A healthy sense of humour adds tremendously to your sex appeal. It's most attractive if you can laugh about yourself, but don't put yourself down too much. If you're a blonde for instance (never mind whether real or fake), tell a silly joke about blondes, and you will see that men relax and are more comfortable chatting to you.*

3 Self-assuredness *The times when a woman was encouraged to be shy and meek are* definitely over. Of course men still love to be admired, but by a woman who is adorable herself. There might be the odd guy out there who finds a weak girl, who needs a strong shoulder to lean on attractive, but most guys prefer a woman who stands on her own feet. It's more and more important for a girl to radiate a healthy amount of self-confidence to be sexually attractive.

4 Sexy Outfit *Erotic attraction isn't just about catching a partner, it's about keeping him or her as well. Staying sexually attractive for each other is a vital part of every relationship and a sexy outfit is usually a winner.*

Men aren't too impressed by all the new trends of couture fashion. They still love to see a woman in a skirt and high heels. The belly-top trend can be very sexy, but only if you don't have too much of a belly and keep your body in great shape. When it comes to underwear, erotic lingerie still takes centre stage. Girls often think they look cute wearing their lover's shirts or boxers, while men have completely different preferences. Black lace lingerie scores the most points with guys. A special treat is a garter belt with stockings, combined with matching bra and panties. It is certain to get a very positive response. It might sound a bit old-fashioned, but when it comes to sexiness this outfit simply can't be beaten.

'I got my girlfriend some sexy lingerie for Christmas,' grins Harry (26) from Co. Kildare. 'A string tanga, bra, garter belt; all in black with red lace trimming. She first refused to wear them for me, saying it would look sluttish. But I convinced her to at least try them on. When she did she looked absolutely fabulous – I had to seduce her on the spot.'

5 Irresistible Smile *It's hard to resist a winning smile. A happy beaming face is much more beautiful and sexy than an unsmiling one. But you need to get your smile just right. Don't flash your teeth like a fake movie star or an eager car salesman. Instead, try to give your smile a mysterious touch. Be careful not to put too much feeling into a smile if you don't really mean to, this could get misunderstood as a promise for more pleasures to come.*

What Makes A Man Sexy?

1 Erotic Body Language Women love to see a man who carries himself self-confidently, comfortable in his body and moving with grace. Not many guys get this right, most move rather awkwardly whether they are in their tracksuit or dressed up in some formal attire.

Try this: when facing a woman, lean forward towards her in an open posture to indicate your attentiveness and interest. Rest a hand languidly on your upper leg, near enough to your privates, but not quite touching them. Don't gesticulate wildly to draw attention to yourself. The more relaxed and confident your gestures and movements are, the sexier you will appear in the woman's eyes.

2 Irresistible Smile An irresistible smile is the surest way into a woman's heart. If you are not sure how to get it right take one of the current heart-throbs as an example. Smile at yourself in a mirror, even if you feel a bit idiotic. Practice until you manage to get the right mix of boyish, seductive and mysterious.

3 Protective Instinct It just feels good to have a shoulder to lean on. So it's no wonder that even the most independent women still seek out men who radiate a strong protective instinct. It makes them feel secure. Women don't go for protective, caring men for any overt logical reason. It's more like a gut feeling they can't resist.

'I regard myself as a career woman; I'm financially independent and have my own life. But I have to admit that I'm longing to find a man whom I can depend on. I've always gone for the protective types and I will keep trying until I find the right one.' Helen (27) from Co. Dublin

4 Fascinating Eyes The eyes are thought to be the mirror of our souls. A look can be anything from bone-chilling to so erotic it flushes you with emotion. There is this old saying that a man can seduce a woman solely with his eyes. It's not too far from the truth. Women can be captivated when a man masters the art of expressing romantic feelings through his eyes. Get it right and your lover will melt in your arms, under your loving gaze.

5 Charisma Charisma is a person's power to attract or influence people. If you want to be more charismatic paying close attention to your appearance is crucial. But it's important not to go overboard. Here are a few helpful hints to get you noticed: don't overdo the shaving; work out to keep your *body in shape; dress casually, but smartly to discreetly show off your assets. Nonchalance, independence and a touch of masculine roughness are your keys to success. It can even help to be a little bit of a selfish bastard to increase your sexy rating in this category.*

'I just love it when a guy looks smart, but a bit rough,' tells Carol (32) from Co. Wicklow. 'At weekends, I don't let my man shave; he is so sexy with dark stubble on his chin. And I absolutely love the smell of him after making love; his fresh sweat is a huge turn on. He keeps teasing me about it, saying I must have animalistic instincts.'

SEX DICTIONARY

EROTIC
Sexually stimulating, regarding to sexual love.

EROTIC ATTRACTION
Awakening sexual interest in another person.

SEX PHEROMONE
A chemical produced by the body to transmit messages to others by means of smell. Sex pheromones are also produced artificially. Artificial pheromones are supposed to increase your sexual attrac-tiveness, but it is very doubtful whether they are effective.

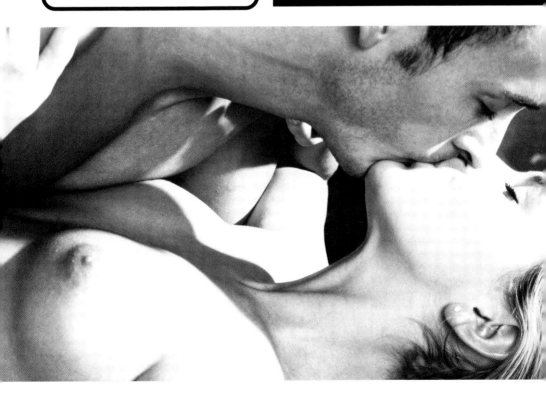

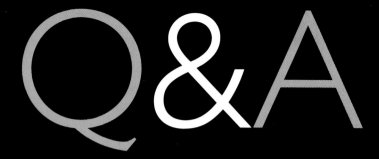

If you feel attracted to somebody on the spot, does that mean that you are meant for each other?

Sexual attraction at first sight is no promise of a happy life together. It's a good start for sure, but only time will tell whether you are meant for each other.

My lover made a great effort to be attractive and charming when I first met him more than a year ago. He looked after himself, went to the gym and dressed smartly. That is all gone now. He has put on weight and looks sloppy. What can I do to return him to his old self?

It looks like he takes you for granted. Many girls and guys make the mistake of letting themselves go once they've found a steady partner. Both sides should make an effort to stay sexually attractive for each other; otherwise the relationship is at risk. Try to coax your lover back into the gym, and then praise him for every gram of fat that he turns into muscle.

I get an erection every time I see this girl. It doesn't happen with others, only with her, although I haven't even spoken to her yet.

That's called erotic attraction. You can feel attracted to somebody at first sight, just by your first glimpse of them. So what happened to you is absolutely normal, there is no need to worry.

My husband has lost all sexual interest in me. I have put on a lot of weight since we met. But then, so has he, and I don't mind. Shouldn't he also accept me the way I am?

You can't force sexual attraction. Why don't you try to get back in shape? It's not only for the sake of your marriage, but also for your personal well-being and general health. Try a new diet, and treat yourself to a make over. I'm sure that you can win your husband's interest back.

My girlfriend is constantly on a diet, claiming she wants to get into shape for me. But I loved her the way she was when we first met. I still love her, but I have gone off her physically since she has become scrawny.

Your girlfriend has to understand that she doesn't do you or herself any favours if she keeps slimming, on the contrary. Remind her that you fell in love with her the way she was when you first met. It is important that you talk openly about this, especially as you don't feel physically attracted to her anymore.

The attractant I spent a small fortune on doesn't work. I seem to be as invisible and undesirable as ever. Is the stuff useless, or should I keep trying?

Some attractants show slight effects, but mainly in laboratory tests only. Under normal conditions, those substances are normally ineffective. If you want women to notice you, there are much better ways to achieve this. Just spraying some sexy scent on you won't do the trick. First of all, make sure you look good and feel confident. Studying the mysteries of body language would help as well.

Why do only the wrong women feel attracted to me? Don't I look the same to all of them?

Your attractiveness not only depends on how you look – you have to take into account how your opponent sees you. If you attract the wrong type of woman, check out what type of guys your ideal girl hangs out with. Observe how they dress and behave, then see whether you'd like to be part of their crowd. If yes, change your outfit to match theirs and see what happens.

I often feel sexually attracted to guys whom I'd never want to have a serious relationship with. Is there any explanation for that?

Sexual attraction and our ideals for the perfect partner don't always go hand in hand. Sexual attraction depends on many factors that we aren't even aware of, like ancient instincts or an unnoticeable pheromone smell. We choose a partner for life much more consciously, weighing up his pros and cons against each other.

Do I have any chance with a pretty girl, although I'm not good looking myself?

Sure, when it comes to sexual attractiveness it's not only beauty that counts, your posture, your charisma, your sense of style and many other factors are important as well. So there is no need to be shy around pretty girls, you have a fair chance if you present yourself the right way.

The guy I fancy doesn't even notice me, although I'm the prettiest girl in our crowd. I've done all I could think of to get his attention, but he completely ignores me.

Maybe you have tried too hard to get this guy's attention. The best approach is to try and impress him in a subtle way, without seeming to be eager.

3 Flirting

What is the secret of being irresistible? It's not your good looks, or the flashy car keys you're rattling or your immaculate styling and outfit. Sure, looking great and driving fancy wheels won't hurt, but it's not your ticket to erotic success. Being a fabulous flirt does the trick.

Flirting is all about the art of being charming, adorable and breathtaking at first sight. You don't have to look stunning to be enticing, but you need to master the art of catching your prey's attention within the first 20 seconds of your first encounter to be a smashing success. What follows is the game of captivating him or her. Once you've got them under your spell the battle is half won.

So far so good, but is there anything you can do to enhance your chances, or is it a question of either you have it, or you don't? No doubt there are some fortunate men and women who are gifted with a natural talent for turning heads and melting hearts, but the humble rest of us need to make some effort to get noticed.

'It used to drive me mad,' confesses Ed (28). 'Some blokes just waltz in blinking an eye, and the finest women start wriggling on their seats all blushed and excited. You look at the guys and can't see what's so special about them. I'm not doing too bad myself nowadays, but it took me years to work out how I can make myself more popular with women.'

There are many unwritten rules you have to follow to be successful. Boasting and showing off won't work. What counts most is your appearance, your body language and attentiveness. If you think it's not worth the hassle, keep in mind that on average, one out of every five serious flirts end up in bed.

Always stick to the rules of good flirting to ensure that there's no rude awakening the next morning. After all, it shouldn't be all about getting laid whatever the costs and circumstances. It's much more fun to meet, attract and love the right one, and it's not that hard to accomplish. But flirting is not only about meeting and conquering somebody new. If you're bound already, it's vital to keep flirting with your partner to keep up the erotic fascination that first drew you to each other. And of course there's nothing wrong with a bit of harmless flirting outside your relationship. It keeps your endorphins flowing – making you happy, content and more fun to be with. So in the end, it keeps your partner much happier as well.

The most obvious places to meet new people are pubs, discos and night-clubs, where drink flows galore and folk are out for the craic. Catching up with the popularity of public watering holes are private parties, which isn't such a big surprise. You're with a crowd of your friends, drinks are much cheaper, and you can even have a smoke without being sent out the door.

The increasing popularity of the work place as a flirting ground is the biggest surprise. One out of every three people consider the work place as one of the best locations for flirting. So work can be much more fun now, it's up to you! There is no doubt that an atmosphere crackling with eroticism can turn a dull working day into a pleasurable experience.

'Since I have started my new job, it is fun being at work,' explains Ellen (28). 'I am the only woman in the place. First the guys weren't too happy to see me joining the team, but now the atmosphere is great. I flirt a bit with most of the lads; it's all harmless and just for fun. But it's more serious with one of them. It's getting hotter between us by the day. We are still at the stage of longing glances and fleeting touches, and it might never go any further, but it still makes it much easier to get up and go to work every morning.'

So let's see how you can hone your flirting skills to perfection. It can't hurt, even if you are a smash hit already.

The Rules of Flirting

1 Dress to Impress

When you meet somebody new, the first 20 seconds will determine your path to success. So make sure you look smart and radiant when you go out. Your best shot is to dress trendy, but please don't go for a posh outfit just for the sake of it. If it doesn't suit you at all forget about it. It would only make you look ridiculous and score against you. Try to develop a trendy but suitable style of your own to stand out in a crowd. Check in front of a mirror to make sure your outfit compliments your body's best assets, be it your bum, your legs, your bosom, whatever is most attractive. Then brighten up your face with an irresistible smile.

2 Smile Don't Snarl

A heart-warming smile is like an open invitation for flirting. To make the smile on your face work wonders, you need to get it right. It won't do to just raise the corners of your lips. Showing your teeth like a shark won't work either. A genuine, whole-hearted smile has to spread all over your face. Such a smile is not only contagious, it will make others relax and feel comfortable in your presence.

3 Get Caught Looking

Look at your object of desire until you get caught looking. Hold the other's gaze for just a split second too long before you allow your eyes to wander languidly over your flirt's body for an initial tantalising check up, taking in every detail. Return your gaze to their face. If your flirt is interested, he or she will seek your eyes again, so be prepared to use that moment to capture your prey. Hold their gaze with the most winning and hypnotising smile you can muster, and the first round goes to you.

4 Be Amusing

Try to be funny and amusing in a quiet and pleasant way without taking over to play the sole entertainer. Be careful with what you joke about, especially if you don't know much about your prey's background and preferences.

Never make embarrassing fun of other people who are there. It might be rewarded with a good laugh, but counts against you in terms of sensitivity. Crack a joke about yourself to show you're only 'lovably' human after all. Try to find out what your flirt finds funny. You might remember a few punch lines of their favourite funny programme. We all love people who resemble ourselves, who share our interests and preferences. To detect a bit of yourself in others makes you feel bonded in a natural way. So once you have found some common ground, you're on your way to success.

5 Start with Fleeting Touches
Once you have established your mutual interest in each other, it is time to carefully move on from the verbal stage of flirting to the first physical contact. Start with fleeting, unobtrusive touches to sociably acceptable areas like the other's arms, back and shoulders. Don't rush upon the sexy zones you can't wait to lay your hands on, as eagerness is one of the worst turn offs in the flirting game. Women should be very careful. Overly friendly touches are misleading signals that can lead to misunderstandings and sometimes trouble.

6 Get the Green Light
Don't spoil your chances by being too keen. Make sure your opposite is interested in you as well before you proceed with your flirting efforts. If your object of desire shows you the cold shoulder, there is no point in making a move. After all, flirting should be fun, not frustrating. Sure, there's some tough folk out there playing hard to get, but your best chance to conquer them is by playing it cool yourself. So make sure the object of your desire shares your interest before you proceed. This also significantly decreases the risk of making a laughing stock of yourself.

This especially goes for men, as women can be very rude and cruel when an unwanted suitor starts getting on their nerves.

7 Be an Attentive Listener
Don't talk too much. Show you care by listening intently to your flirt. Invite your opposite to talk about themselves. Ask questions that show your earnest interest, but aren't too intrusive. Chat about films, music or other hobbies to find some area of mutual interest. Reign the course of your conversation, but let the other do most of the talking. It's your chance to make an impression by proving yourself to be a good and attentive listener.

8 Make Realistic Compliments
Women and men alike fish for compliments to lift their self-esteem. So don' be stingy with compliments, dish them out. To make a compliment work, it has to be at least basically realistic. You can't charm Miss Average by telling her she looks like Miss World. Compliments need to be credible to be appreciated and savoured, so compliment your flirt on their best assets. That can be long legs, a sexy bum, nice hair, lovely eyes, or one of a hundred other features. Try to find out what your flirt is most proud of. It's normally not hard to tell if you keep your eyes open, as most people make it pretty obvious by advertising it themselves.

9 Be Gentle If You Reject Somebody

It's a real pain to be approached by the wrong person, especially when the right one is present as well. As you well know from your own feelings, nobody wants to be rejected, so do it as gently as possible if it needs to be done. Even if you can't wait to get rid of an unwanted candidate, you have to stay as friendly and gentle as the situation allows. Never make fun of somebody who's approached you, and avoid being rude. It's not only unkind towards your unlucky suitor, but it would keep others from trying their luck.

10 Make Body Language Work For You

Your body language reveals much more about yourself than you are probably aware of. For somebody who keeps their eyes open and who knows how to interpret the signs, your appearance, movements, and posture give away your mood, your character, and much more.

Body language plays a vital role in the flirting game, so knowing how to interpret the signs definitely improves your flirting skills. You can read your opposite like an open book, and discover and nip any setbacks in your flirting process in the bud. You can also ensure that you send out the right and most encouraging signals yourself.

The most promising posture is if your prey leans over towards you, with their arms held openly, and their hands either relaxed or gently caressing a sensitive, but not too obviously erotic spot on their body, like the inside of the upper leg. Another encouraging sign is if you catch her or him mirroring your own posture or gestures. If she or he starts rubbing their leg a split second after you've started to rub your own, or raise their drink after you've just taken a sip yourself, that's a strong signal of interest.

Practice your own body language before you go out. Never flirt looking defensive, with your legs clenched and your arms wrapped tightly across your chest. You'll never catch your dream partner's attention if you're sending out the wrong signals. Keep an open posture, turn towards your prey, mirror their gestures, and see if you can get an encouraging response.

11 Be Spontaneous

Be adventurous and spontaneous to find the best flirting grounds. Don't stick to the traditional meeting places like pubs and nightclubs alone; you'd miss your best chances. There are so many opportunities out there if you only keep your eyes open. All you have to do is be spontaneous and grab your chances, be it on the street, waiting for the bus, out shopping or anywhere else.

12 Scout the Right Places

To find your perfect match, look in the right places. Whether it's walking on the beach, running in the park, or attending an evening class – look where you will most likely bump into someone who shares your interests. Joining a dancing class is a good tip for guys, as women will outnumber them for sure. And dancing is an activity that allows close bodily contact.

Another promising place to flirt is the supermarket. You can easily spend an hour pushing your trolley without looking like a desperate eejit. That gives you plenty of time to wait for somebody tempting to show up. Now imagine all the possibilities a supermarket provides you with. Just park your trolley beside your flirt's, and then drop your shopping into their trolley – by mistake! You don't even have to be the one to speak first, as they will most probably mention it first. Make sure to have a witty response ready to grab the opportunity.

'This is how I met my boyfriend,' explains Linda (25). 'I was out shopping, and this bloke put a chicken into my trolley, right beside the one I had gotten for myself. When I told him it was my trolley not his, he apologised, and pointed out that we obviously have the same taste. Amazingly, he had the same stuff in his trolley: potato wedges, garlic bread, salad, a bottle of white wine – and then the chicken. When I handed it over to him, he asked nonchalantly whether I had any idea how to cook it, as he'd never cooked chicken before. Weeks later he confessed that it had all been a trick to chat me up. And it worked!'

The Rules of Flirting

1 Dress to Impress
2 Smile Don't Snarl
3 Get Caught Looking
4 Be Amusing
5 Start with Fleeting Touches
6 Get the Green Light
7 Be an Attentive Listener
8 Make Realistic Compliments
9 Be Gentle If You Reject Somebody
10 Make Body Language Work For You
11 Be Spontaneous
12 Scout the Right Places

Jealousy

Flirting could be even more fun if it wasn't for jealousy. Even people who love to flirt themselves tend to suffer the nagging feeling of jealousy when they watch their partner flirting.

Are you jealous when you catch your partner flirting?

Always	26%
Most of the time	18%
Depends	35%
Seldom	10%
Never	11%

So one out of four people (26%) are always jealous when they catch their partner flirting with some-body else. Only one out of nine (11%) never suffers from bouts of jealousy. It is not easy to accomplish, but you should at least try to keep your jealousy in check, for your own sake as much as for your partner's.

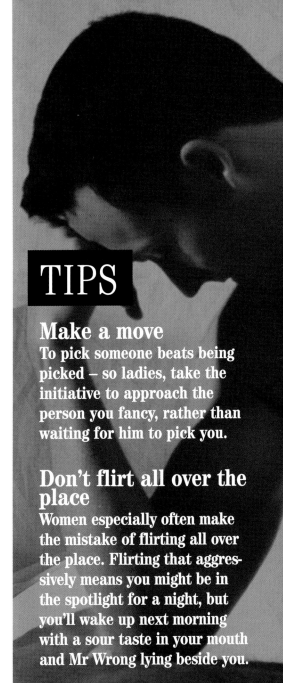

TIPS

Make a move
To pick someone beats being picked – so ladies, take the initiative to approach the person you fancy, rather than waiting for him to pick you.

Don't flirt all over the place
Women especially often make the mistake of flirting all over the place. Flirting that aggressively means you might be in the spotlight for a night, but you'll wake up next morning with a sour taste in your mouth and Mr Wrong lying beside you.

Don't give up
Don't resign if you get rejected. Review your tactics, improve your skills, and keep trying.

SEX DICTIONARY

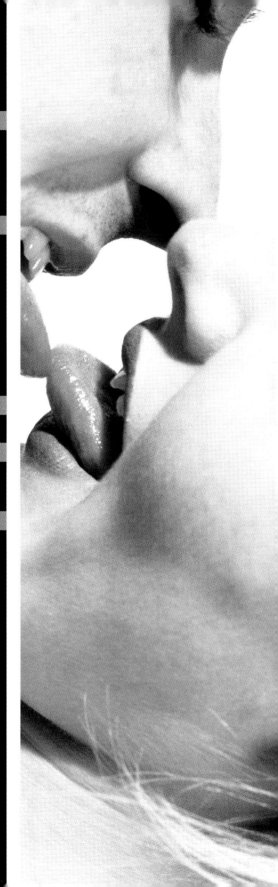

BODY LANGUAGE
The expression of feelings and thoughts not verbally, but by bodily signs, like gestures, postures, and body movement.

ENDORPHIN
A body chemical that serves to suppress pain and can help to achieve an euphoric state, like a natural high. Its production within our body is triggered by a wide range of factors and activities, like stress, danger, physical exercise, and sexual activity.

EROTIC
Sexually stimulating.

FLIRTING
Playful way to make romantic overtures and arouse sexual interest.

MIRRORING TECHNIQUE
Based on the assumption that we feel unconsciously attracted to people who's body language resembles our own, the mirroring technique is a way to make others feel comfortable in our presence, and make them wish to be with us. The basic strategy is to consciously copy the other person's gestures and movements to trigger off their unconscious attraction towards you. Cross your legs when your opposite does, raise your glass when they raise their's, smile when they do.

Q&A

When I go out to a pub or a bar, is there a quick check that allows me to tell which women might be interested in me?

You can tell with a few simple checks whether you might have a chance or not. First of all, look around to see whether any of the women there are looking at you. If you catch a woman eyeing you, give her a smile and see what happens. If she looks away only to meet your eyes again in a second or two – good luck! If she turns her eyes away and avoids looking in your direction again – forget about it. Another quick check is to walk past a woman to force her to notice you, then to sit or stand in her line of vision. If she turns away to face another direction, you've obviously failed to interest her. If she's interested, she will make a move by seeking eye contact.

I am too shy to talk to a girl – How can I make girls talk to me first?

Women are very careful when chatting up shy guys; the risk of being rejected is too high. Of course you can try to lure women over to you by sending out the right signals, but even then: are you sure your shyness would be gone the moment a woman talks to you? I very much doubt that. Better treat this problem by the roots. Visit places where people naturally chat with each other. This can be an evening course, a sports club, voluntarily work for a charity, group holidays – whatever. Being in a free and easy mixed crowd where people share the same interests not only holds lots of relaxed opportunities for flirting, it also gives you a chance to get to know the opposite sex better, which will help you to overcome your shyness.

Why is it that the wrong guys always chat me up?

Most guys wait until they get at least a little bit of encouragement before they chat a girl up. So you must be sending out the wrong signals. An important factor is your appearance. Observe which type of girls the guys you fancy go for. How are they dressed? Do they wear make-up? Are they bubbly flirtatious types or quiet ones? Compare your own appearance and behaviour with theirs, and you will see what you can do to compete with them and get the guys you're after.

Is it okay to flirt with somebody else when I'm in a steady relationship?

There is nothing wrong with flirting while you are in a relationship, as long as you don't go too far. The tingle of flirting lifts your spirits, making you happier and more content. So flirting even has a positive effect on your relationship, as a happy person is more fun to be with. Still, I wouldn't take a flirt too far, as it's not fair on your partner to sleep with others, at least not if you haven't agreed to live in an open relationship where both of you can do as you please.

Is a woman going to be branded a slut if she takes the initiative?

Most guys are open minded enough to appreciate it if a woman makes a move, as long as she's not too bold or appears to be too keen. To make sure you don't ruin your chances it's best not to be too straight forward. Sure, it's unfair, but women still don't get away with all the nasty things men are often allowed to do.

How do I read a woman's body language? What are the signs that tell you not to bother, and which signs are more encouraging? When can I feel safe to go ahead? Keep it simple please!

Don't bother to approach a woman if she looks sullen, lets her head hang down or sits or stands in a defensive posture, clutching herself or turning her back to you. Send out signals to a woman you fancy, smile at her, and try to hold her gaze. If she returns your smiles, keep going. Small gestures like flipping her hair back or absently caressing her own body, are pretty strong signals of interest. If she even bothers to brush past you a couple of times, you can't do much wrong by saying hello. Then, take it from there. Don't be too keen on your first approach, but try to stay relaxed. Wait for the right opportunity to suggest going out together.

4 Expectations – What Makes a Good Lover

One of the most common questions I'm asked is, 'What makes a good lover?' What do we need to have in our repertoire to make sure that we don't disappoint in bed?

Let's look at the essentials. First of all, you have to be trustful. Then you definitely have to be good at kissing. A good lover has to be able to read the other's mind and body language, and respond to it. Sex is best when both partners try to fulfil each other's wishes. They also need to be sensitive, and to react to their partner's slightest signs of pleasure or discomfort.

Both men and women agree that tenderness and passion are other preconditions for good sex but after that it starts to get difficult. Except for the few basics that both sexes agree on, men and women have very different ideas of what makes a good lover.

'A good lover has to be a seducer. He needs to give me the feeling that I am somebody very special for him, and that it's not only sex he is after,' says Barbara (32).

'A woman has to be experienced and know all the tricks to be a good lover. I don't want fumbling, but knowing hands on my body,' says Marcel (26).

We can't project our own wishes and preferences onto a member of the opposite sex. As a woman, you might think that if you master the art of light caressing and stroking, you are a perfect lover. Not so – most men prefer a massaging hand.

Let's shed some light on all the mysteries by clearly showing the different expectations of both sexes.

What Makes A Man A Good Lover?

1 Kissing A good kiss makes a woman melt in your arms. Don't kiss in exactly the same way all the time. Play with her lips and tongue, move from teasing and tender to passionate. Look into her eyes before you close your mouth down over hers for a kiss. You can't go wrong with imitating romantic kissing scenes you have seen in a romantic movie.

2 Caressing and Stroking A good lover has to master the art of caressing and tenderly stroking a woman's body. That's not as easy as it sounds, for caressing has to be done in the right way. It has to be performed with feeling, like you are enjoying it yourself. Just carelessly moving your hands over a woman's body isn't caressing, and it will bring you more criticism than praise.

3 Seducing Seduce your woman even if she is already beside you in bed. Don't take her willingness to make love with you for granted. You have to win her love again and again.

'My husband is great at that,' tells Amy (29). 'He always makes an effort to seduce me. He often starts hours before we go to bed. Sometimes he brings me flowers or he sends a text message or starts massaging my neck and shoulders. Or he invites me to share a bath with him.'

4 Clitoris Massage

There is nothing more annoying than a big rough thumb rubbing on the wrong spot. Clitoris massage is an art that requires a very sensitive hand. It is not good enough to know essentially where to start, you have to sense the slightest signs of pleasure or discomfort your woman shows in order to react to them properly. If you don't know yet what your lover prefers, try light circling caresses around her clitoris, just with a finger or two. In case you can't find the right touch, let her show you what she likes.

5 Delay Orgasm

A lover has to be good at delaying his orgasm, in order to wait for his woman to come first. Once she is ready to come, a perfect lover is able to delay her orgasm as well to prolong her moments of ecstasy. This is a risky game, for the smallest mistake can spoil everything.

6 Oral Sex

One out of every three Irish women (36%) longs for her lover to master oral techniques when making love. You can't go wrong with tenderly licking a woman's clitoris for starters. To improve your technique, you need to find out what your woman likes

best, and there is only one way to achieve that – keep trying and experimenting, and react to any signs of pleasure or discomfort that she shows.

7 Other Essentials

What else does a man need to be good at? Three out of every ten Irish women (30%) expects a good lover to master various positions. Even if she likes the missionary position best, there has to be some variation from time to time to keep lovemaking exciting. A good bit of potency is asked for as well: a really good lover should be able to perform more often than once.

A big surprise from the survey was discovering that one out of every 14 Irish women (7%) wants her lover to be good at bondage. Ruth (42) from Co. Mayo is one of them:

'It drives me mad with desire to let a guy have total control over me. Of course I have to trust him absolutely and I want to talk about how far he is allowed to go. But then, he has to bind my wrists and ankles onto the bedposts, leaving me spread-eagled. He has to be gentle, but firm as well. When he asks something silly, like whether I am comfortable enough, the whole game is spoilt for me.'

What Makes A Woman A Good Lover?

1 Kissing *That good kissing is essential for good love is one of the few points both sexes agree on, although their tastes in kissing aren't exactly the same. Women love tender and romantic kisses, while lads often like it a bit more rough and wet. Women like to play around softly and teasingly, nibbling on lips and tongue, while guys prefer deep kisses with intense tongue contact.*

2 Variety of Positions *Men like a woman to be good at trying out various positions. Irish men especially love the woman to be on top – to spoil them. There are so many variations of that position that trying them all out will keep you busy for a good few nights.*

And there are so many other ways of making love that you can keep busy all your life trying out new variations and angles.

3 Oral Sex *Erotic kisses are an essential part of a good lover's repertoire. Every second Irish man interviewed (50%), said a woman has to be good at spoiling him orally. It is not enough to just apply a few kisses and take the penis into your mouth – all this has to be done right. Although most men are happier if their partner makes at least a shy and rather awkward*

effort, that is not what they really dream of. Men want to be brought to orgasm expertly. The ultimate kick for them is to come in her mouth.

4 Penis Massage *Guys love to be masturbated by a woman, but it needs a good bit of practice to get it right. Most women have too light a grip on the penis, more tickling than massaging it, like they are afraid of hurting it. Women should let their lovers show them how they want to be massaged. If he puts his own hand over hers, she can feel the amount of pressure that needs to be applied, and will also get an idea about which kind of strokes he loves best.*

'My girlfriend touches my penis so lightly that I can hardly feel her hand,' complains Oisin (31). 'I love to feel a firm grip on the penis shaft, and I have already showed her a few times, but she is still afraid that she might hurt me when she gives me a proper squeeze. I always have to put my hand over hers in the end, otherwise I couldn't climax.'

5 **Petting** *A good lover has to be perfect at petting. The main criticism guys come up with is that a woman's touch is too light and fleeting on the penis and that they often squeeze the testicles too heartily. In case you didn't notice yet: men also love to be touched up through their clothes.*

6 **Position 69** *You can't blame men for being selfish when it comes to oral sex. Most men are as eager to give oral pleasures as they are to receive them. Oral sex in perfection is epitomised by position 69. The numbers 6 and 9 illustrate how your bodies should be arranged. More than one out of every three Irish men (36%) expects a woman to master this technique. Once you have overcome the technical hurdles, you'll see that it's worth the effort. It is an exceptional erotic feeling to caress your partner's genitals orally while he does the same to you.*

7 **Other Essentials** *There's no question that sometimes men like being spoiled. They want their lover to know the little tricks and games that give them pleasure. One out of four Irish men (28%) wants his lover to be good at body massage. A good, relaxing body massage gets him into the mood for more, especially if you massage him naked or in a sexy outfit and don't spare the grunts of pleasure and admiration. Every fourth guy (25%) appreciates a lover who can master the skill of verbal erotic or talking dirty, while one out of seven (15%) want a woman to be good at making love to them with her breasts.*

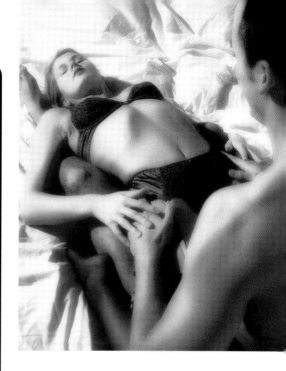

Ireland's Lovers

What Irish Women Want:

Kissing	80%
Caressing, stroking	74%
Seducing	57%
Clitoris massage	40%
Delay orgasm	37%
Oral sex	36%
Variety of positions	30%
Body massage	18%
Petting	16%
Sex several times in a row	14%
Position 69	13%
Games of bondage	7%

What Irish Men Want:

Kissing	60%
Variety of positions	52%
Oral sex	50%
Penis massage	42%
Petting	37%
Position 69	36%
Caressing	32%
Seducing	31%
Body massage	28%
Sex several times in a row	27%
Verbal sex	25%
Sex between the breasts	15%

That Loving Feeling –
What conditions do you need for good sex?

	Women	Men
Trust	94%	90%
Tenderness	83%	80%
Passion	58%	74%
Naturalness	54%	44%
Love to Experiment	37%	63%

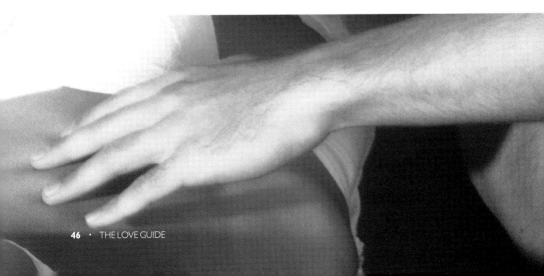

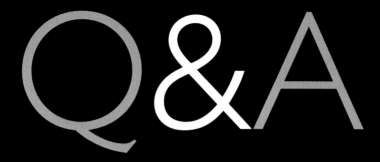

Q&A

My new boyfriend can't get erect again right after he has had his orgasm. It takes him at least 20 minutes, and I can't wait that long.

The time a man needs to become physically aroused again after his orgasm differs from a couple of minutes to a couple of hours, so your boyfriend isn't doing too badly if it takes him only 20 minutes. If you can't wait that long, ask him to keep you aroused using his hands and lips in the meantime.

When in bed with my lover I don't get half of what I want. Is it okay for a woman to take charge of lovemaking, or should I take it as it comes?

Of course it is okay for a woman to take charge. If you don't get what you want, it's probably because your partner simply doesn't know what you fancy. So show him. Take over the reins and make love to him the way you like it, I'm sure he won't complain.

My husband sexually neglects me; he makes love to me only once or twice per month. Should I sleep with another man?

I can't see what good sleeping with another man would do to your marriage. Before you go on any adventures try to get your marriage back on track first. Try to seduce your husband by snuggling up to him and touching him intimately. If he doesn't respond to your efforts, talk to him.

For my girlfriend it is not enough to make love once, I always have to perform a second time. When I don't manage, she gets annoyed and accuses me of being selfish. How can I satisfy her?

Make sure your girlfriend has an orgasm before you come yourself. Spoil her with a long foreplay, and then try to stimulate her clitoris manually while you make love to her. That demands a bit of patience, but it saves you the second go that you dread so much.

My partner doesn't know anything about sex. The worst is the way she kisses me intimately. I don't know what to do about this. Every time I show her that I'm displeased, she starts crying.

Your partner obviously tries to please you, so it is only normal that she is disappointed when you let her feel that her efforts aren't good enough for you. Instead of being annoyed, you should be understanding and patient. Appreciate her efforts, and show her, in a loving way, how you like being touched and kissed. And don't forget to spoil her sexually as well.

I know this is a bit unusual for a woman, but I love to talk dirty when we make love. My new boyfriend wants me to stop it. Our love life could be much nicer if he'd play along. How can I make him understand?

Try a compromise. He can't expect you to shut up in bed, but you could at least refrain from using obscene language, as vulgarity obviously turns him off. Talk sexy instead of dirty, and your boyfriend might even learn to enjoy it.

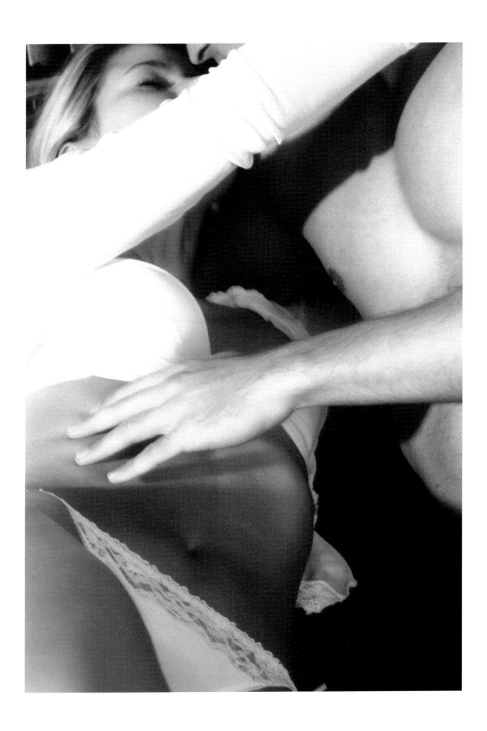

5 Erotic Fantasies

Did you ever have an erotic fantasy in the most inappropriate situation? For instance, were you ever in a boring meeting at work and all of a sudden a juicy, erotic fantasy popped into your mind? Or were you ever in a club and in your mind's eye you start stripping the gorgeous looking creature you have only just met?

If yes, you are in good company. Our survey revealed that erotic fantasies play a huge role in Irish people's everyday life. Women as well as men, experience sexual fantasies anytime, whenever they feel like it. It can be during a walk in the park, in a traffic jam, while they are chatting with somebody – more or less any occasion and any circumstance will do. The locations and occasions are countless. Fantasies occur much more often than most of us would think: on average, Irish people have at least one erotic fantasy per day, with men fantasising more often than women.

Most of the time, erotic fantasies just pop up out of the blue, when we see something that turns us on, think about somebody special, or for no apparent reason at all. At other times, we start our fantasies purposefully to arouse and entertain ourselves.

We often start fantasising when we are with our partner, and need something extra to turn us on and get our hormones flowing. And of course we produce sexual fantasies galore while we are masturbating, to spice up this do-it-yourself-act.

There are many ways to stimulate erotic fantasies. For women, romantic music works best, while men strongly react to sexy lingerie. For those who don't have much experience with sexual fantasies themselves, erotic pictures and films are helpful to give them the right ideas and to get their imagination going.

Most of us (93%) rate their sexual fantasies as normal, while seven per cent describe them as sick or perverse. Where normal erotic fantasies end and perverse ones start, varies from one person to the next. What one person might consider a normal fantasy another might find disgusting or even perverse.

'My first husband used to dream about dressing up in black domina gear, and then using a whip on my naked bum. He found that fantasy normal, while I still think it is perverse.' Helga (52) from Co. Wexford.

We keep most of our fantasies to ourselves. Only one out of every five Irish people (21%) often shares their erotic fantasies with their partner. But another six out of ten of us (61%) discuss at least some of their sex fantasies with their better half. It is important to talk about your sexual fantasies. There might be one or two that your partner would like to share with you.

Kevin (34) from Co. Meath explains: 'It depends what I am fantasising about. When it's something we can live out together, like making love on a mountain peak, I share the fantasy with my wife. But I can hardly tell her that I dream of having kinky sex with Madonna.'

Three out of every four Irish couples (73%) make at least some of their fantasies come true by playing them out together.

Who takes part in sexual fantasies?

Apart from their own partner, women mainly fantasise about another man they have once been in love with – their ex. It's no wonder that women keep so many of their fantasies secret. No guy would be pleased to know that his beloved still dreams of her ex.

'I can't help but fantasise about him,' explains Janet (26) from Co. Kerry. 'He was my first lover, and we were a perfect match in bed. Even when I sleep with my husband now, I often fantasise about my first love being with me again.'

More than one out of five Irish women (23%) enjoy forbidden fantasy encounters with the film star of their dreams. This type of fantasy man is much less threatening, as he's a total stranger. One out of every four women (25%) dreams of intimate encounters with Mr Unknown and one out of six (16%) has erotic fantasies about a friend.

Irish men fantasise mainly about sexual encounters with their partner (53%). In second place are fantasies about total strangers (35%) and not too far behind are friends: three out of ten guys (30%) thinks erotically about a friend. This highlights the point that it is really difficult for men to stay 'friends only' with a woman. In fourth place is a younger partner, closely followed by an ex-partner.

'Although I am 36 myself, I still love young women around twenty. Especially when I masturbate, I don't think of my wife, but fantasise about much younger women. I let them touch and kiss me in my dreams, and have them strip off to show their young bodies.' Ben (36) from Co. Dublin.

What takes place in sexual fantasies?

Women's sexual fantasies are mainly about tenderness (43%). Fantasies about sex on the beach take an astonishing second place (39%), closely followed by romantic encounters in general (36%).

'Sex on the beach is one of my favourite fantasies,' tells Moira (48) from Co. Galway, 'but I would never dream of putting it into reality. It is fantastic, romantic, and very erotic as it is: as a mere fantasy. I dream of making love to my favourite singer on the beach. Why should I spoil that fantasy by trying to live it out with my completely unromantic husband?'

For men, oral sex is the most often mentioned part of their sexual fantasies (53%). But tenderness is important for males as well: four out of ten Irish men (39%) dream about lots of tenderness in their erotic fantasies, and one out of three (34%) fantasises about having a threesome. Sex on the beach plays an important role in every third man's fantasies (33%), but in a less romantic context.

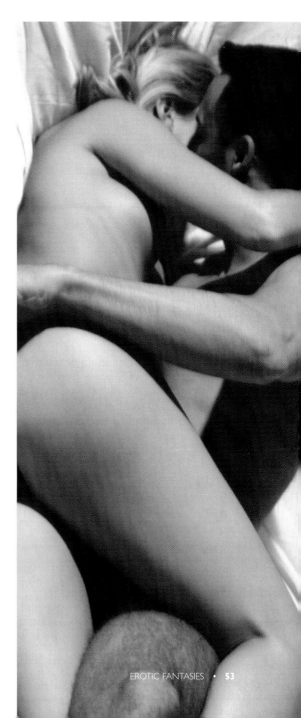

The survey revealed that an astonishing three out of every ten men (30%) fantasise about having sex in a car. Most of them dream about a woman spoiling them with fellatio. Others don't have their own car in mind, but a comfortable limousine, as Brian (31) from Co. Louth describes in his hottest dream:

'I got the idea from a film. A woman was being chauffeured to a function in her rich lover's stretch limousine, and she invited this young guy in. They had a great time making love in the huge backseat, coursing through the streets.'

In the multiple-choice survey hundreds of Irish people were asked the following questions:

When Do You Have Sexual Fantasies?

	Total
I just fit them in when I feel like it, like at work	35%
When I masturbate	33%
When I am with my partner and need an extra turn on	23%
When I can't fulfil my sexual wishes	22%
When my sex life is getting boring	17%

Who Takes Part In Your Sexual Fantasies?

	Women	Men
My partner	69%	53%
Total strangers	25%	35%
Friends	16%	30%
Ex-partner	27%	24%
Somebody younger than me	10%	25%
Film stars	23%	15%
Rock or pop stars	16%	12%
Colleagues	7%	17%
Somebody older/and more experienced	12%	11%
TV celebrities	5%	12%

What Takes Place in Your Sexual Fantasies?

	Women	Men
Cheating	15%	31%
Lots of tenderness	43%	39%
Scenes from books, magazines or newspapers	33%	18%
Romantic encounters	36%	22%
Oral sex	30%	53%
Caressing of breasts	34%	32%
Threesome	17%	34%
Sex on the beach	39%	33%
Sex games in the car	22%	30%
Sex with strangers	13%	22%

A Few Fantasies

Women *I am standing naked at an open window. Everybody can look inside but only one guy notices me. While he stares in at me, I slowly start touching myself. First I caress my breasts, then my hand moves down between my legs, while he is still watching me.*

I am on the beach. I ask this great looking guy to put some sun lotion on my back. He starts slowly to rub it in. His hands move all over my back, then my upper legs and my bum, caressing me. He slips his hand under my belly, and in between my legs to slowly caress me there.

Men *My female colleague walks into the office in the nude. She comes over to me and starts to kiss my lips, while her hands go to work on the buttons of my shirt and the zipper of my trousers. She seduces me right there on the desk. Other people could walk in at any time.*

I am in bed with my girlfriend, asleep. When I wake up, I feel her lips around my penis, and her hands gently massaging my testicles.

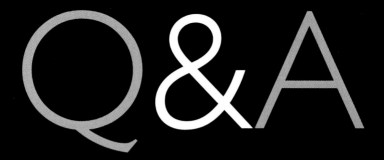

Q&A

Is it okay to fantasise about another man when I sleep with my guy? Or should I feel guilty?

There is nothing wrong with fantasising about somebody else when you sleep with your guy, it's pretty normal. Just be aware that he might be fantasising about somebody else as well. Talk to each other and you could get your longings and wishes in sync.

I would love to see my boyfriend ejaculate when we make love. My fantasy of watching him come drives me mad with desire. I even dream about it. The problem is that I'm afraid to tell him about my sexual wish. Isn't it best to keep this desire to myself?

No, absolutely not. If you want to watch your boyfriend ejaculate, tell him how much this fantasy turns you on – he might find it exciting himself. If you are too shy to talk about it, try to make him come with your hands and lips. I'm sure he won't mind.

My husband doesn't show much interest in sex anymore. He is always tired or has other things on his mind. I'm very frustrated about this, and have come to the conclusion that I have to do something about it. My fantasy is to try out sex with two men. One of them could be my husband, the other one an open minded, adventurous lad. I have this fantasy more and more often, but I'm not sure how to present it to my husband.

The best way to introduce your husband to your idea is to talk about it in a casual way first to check out what he thinks about it, but I'm afraid he won't be enthusiastic about your dream of sharing the marriage bed with another guy. Irrespective of your wish to try out a threesome, you should talk to your husband about what's lacking in your relationship from your point of view. He might not even be aware of the fact that you feel neglected.

My girlfriend and I have fantasies about going nude on the beach. Is there an organisation called the Irish Naturist Association that organise weekend breaks together? Could you give us some information about this organisation?

There is an Irish Naturist Association (INA) that promotes Naturism in Ireland. They can provide you with information about nudist beaches at home and abroad. During the summer, they often organise events, or just meet informally on the beach - weather permitting. Contact: The Irish Naturist Association, PO Box 1077, Churchtown, Dublin 14, Ireland. Phone: 086-837 0395 Fax: 086-5837 0395 Web: http://www.esatclear.ie/~irishnaturist/

I have sexual dreams and fantasies that are upsetting and even frightening me. When I married my husband I was still a virgin, and I have always been faithful to him since. Now all of a sudden I dream of having wild nights with total strangers, of dressing up sexily and seducing younger guys, and even of taking part in unusual sex games. Most of all, I feel a strong urge to cheat on my husband to find out what it would be like with another man. The worst is that I feel like my best years are nearly over and I'm running out of time. I don't know what got into me but whatever it is, my disturbing fantasies are a matter of serious concern to me.

For a woman who was married young and inexperienced, and has had sex with only one man all her life, your sexual fantasies aren't at all unusual. Being with the same man since adolescence, you can't help wondering whether maybe you are missing out on something. Approaching a more mature stage of your life, you are worried that you might never be able to catch up with whatever you might be missing if you don't do it now. The best way to get through this crisis unharmed is to seriously spice up your marital sex life. Dress up sexily to seduce your husband, surprise him with the sex games that you've been fantasising about.

Recently I found out that my cousin is a lesbian. When I think about it, I get really aroused, and I want to ejaculate every night before I go to sleep. I even get images of her in my head to help me come a lot quicker. Does this mean I have feelings for my cousin?

Don't mistake sexual interest for love. Your fantasies don't mean that you have any feelings for your cousin. They merely show that her being a lesbian turns you on immensely. This is not unusual. Most men use sexual fantasies when they masturbate and the idea of lesbian love is one of the most arousing.

When I sleep with my husband, I always have very strong romantic fantasies. Sometimes I imagine us in a big four-poster in some fancy hotel room or I think about sexual adventures we had in the past. I feel guilty about what I'm doing but it is the only way I can enjoy sex.

Don't feel bad about your fantasies. They help you to enjoy your sex life, and there is nothing wrong with that. But why not put some fantasies into reality? Don't wait for your husband to take the initiative. You know what you fancy, so go for it. Most men are more than happy when their wife takes over the initiative and gives them a taste of what they desire.

There is a fantasy that I can't stop thinking about. My wife has fabulous breasts. They are big but firm and well-shaped. I would love so much to come on her breasts but every time I try, she tells me that she needs to feel me inside her.

Tell your wife how much her breasts turn you on. Next time you sleep with her, make sure she gets an orgasm while you are inside her. Then pull out before you climax yourself, and ask her whether it's okay if you come on her breasts for a change.

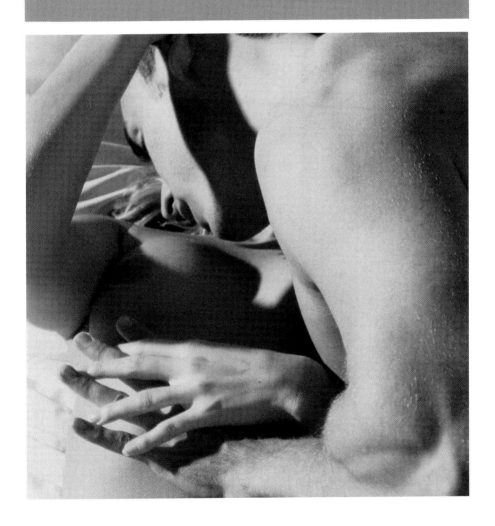

6 Foreplay

Foreplay is, or ideally should be, the starting point of an intimate encounter. It doesn't always have to lead to intercourse but most couples see it as a warm-up phase that allows your body and mind to get into the right mood for the pleasures to come.

The physical side of foreplay basically gets your sexual organs lubricated and ready for action. For men, this only takes a few minutes, while women take much longer to get prepared for intercourse.

The average foreplay lasts for 24 minutes, with huge deviations in both directions. Some couples don't bother with foreplay at all, while others spend an hour or more on kissing and teasing before they sleep together. While most men are more than content with the duration of their foreplay, women generally wish for a bit more.

It is not only important how much time you spend on foreplay, but how you spend this time. A very special treat is to kiss your partner from top to toe, especially if you concentrate on his or her personal erogenous zones even though they might not have much appeal for you, like her back or his feet. Don't leave out the genital zone. Men especially would be badly disappointed or even frustrated if after you spent half an hour kissing him all over, working around his most sensitive spots, you stopped without giving him the ultimate pleasure.

To spice up your foreplay, you can use sexy lingerie, sex toys, erotic books or movies, play sex games – it's up to you and whatever fantasy works for you. The most important thing is to get your partner and yourself into the right mood. Women, on average, take much longer than men to get sexually aroused. To be on the safe side, check whether her vagina is moist enough for you to slip in comfortably, using your hand or the tip of your penis. Don't try to penetrate a dry vagina; it's like trying to break through a brick wall. It is uncomfortable and sometimes painful for both parties, leaving you both sore and frustrated. This can easily be avoided by having a bit more patience or by simply applying a lubricant. If you don't have a lubricant at hand, use saliva, which can be applied by tongue and lips.

Five Foreplay Favourites

1 Passionate Kisses

Passionate kisses are the perfect start for foreplay. Let your tongue and teeth play with your partner's lips and tongue. Caress, nibble gently, and tease. Stroke his or her cheeks and temples while you kiss, put your hands into their hair to gently rub their scalp. When your kiss gets deeper, let your partner feel your body press against them. Let your hands glide over their body, exploring, stroking, caressing or lightly squeezing. Start at the shoulders, then languidly stroke down their back, moving your hands slowly down towards the buttocks.

2 Caressing the Genitals

Who doesn't like to get their genitals caressed by a loving hand? In foreplay, it's important that you don't start on the genitals straight away. Before you concentrate on them, take your time to make your partner's body more sensitive by caressing less obvious areas of pleasure. Touch the inner thighs, trace the lines of his or her loins with your fingertips, playfully tease the delicate, sensitive skin all around the most private places, before you move over to the genitals themselves.

Let your partner show you the best spots to give them ultimate pleasure and how they like to get touched there.

3 Caressing the Breasts

Men as well as women love getting their chests caressed but you have to be very careful how you do it, especially when you have a go at your partner's nipples.

Only ten per cent of Irish women and nine per cent of Irish men like to get their nipples pinched, gently nibbled or softly bitten. Sucking isn't really popular either. The only caress that is enjoyed by almost everybody, men and women alike, is gentle stroking. Tender kisses take second stage, followed by licking. Everything that goes beyond these gentle caresses has to be checked out carefully before you go ahead. But it's worth checking; otherwise you might be missing out on pleasures that both you and your partner fancy, but that you're afraid to try out.

'I love it when my man strokes and kisses my breasts, but he has to be very careful when he gets near my nipples,' explains Ellen (24). 'Sometimes it feels great when he gently bites or sucks them, while most of the time they are too sensitive but I don't know about that until he tries.'

4 Oral Kisses *Oral kisses are the best way to drive your partner mad with desire and to spoil him or her. Women like very gentle but then more urgent licking of their clitoris. The most appreciated technique is to move your tongue around the clitoris in circular movements. It takes some practise to find out the exact amount of pressure and tempo you need to apply.*

To please a man orally is a bit easier. Let your lips and tongue play with the top of his penis, then take him into your mouth. Move your lips up and down upon his penis and try to simultaneously tease him with your tongue.

You can't go far wrong with that, as long as you are careful not to scratch his delicate skin with your teeth.

Teasing All Over

5 *Teasing is the new art of foreplay. It is all about driving each other mad with desire. Light and fleeting touches in your sensitive areas make you tingle with desire and expectation – making you lust for more. Caress your partner's back, lightly scratch their inner thighs and gently trace the line of their loins with your fingertip or your tongue. Never hurry. For good teasing you need to take all the time in the world.*

'My lover is a master of teasing. He drives me mad with his foreplay, first kissing my whole body, and then letting the tip of his penis play around my clitoris for ages until I can't stand to be without him any longer. I literally have to beg him to get inside me. Normally I come the very moment he thrusts himself in.' Marion (25)

'My husband is great at teasing me. On a Sunday morning, he serves me breakfast in bed, with fresh fruit and cream, the whole lot. We eat the fruit off each other's bodies, from my belly-button, my breasts, and his penis. We always end up making passionate love.' Rhonda (31)

There are many ways to tease your lover, but there are a couple of recipes that hardly ever fail to work:

To Tease HER

Start playing with her lips. Gently nibble her upper lip and then trace the inside of her lips with the tip of your tongue while you hold her in a loose embrace. Keep teasing her lips with your tongue until your kiss becomes more urgent and passionate.

Move your hands over her back and bum, then let your hand move between her legs, but only to retreat again, then make another move and start caressing her clitoris. Concentrate on what you're doing. When you feel she's ready to come, hold back a little bit more. Fool around with the tip of your penis at the entrance of her vagina for what should feel like forever, until she begs you to enter her. Don't give in too quickly, but prolong this game until both of you can't stand it any longer.

To Tease HIM

Grab his genitals through his pants to make him grow. Gently squeeze and caress him through the fabric. Don't let him open his pants until you allow him to do so.

Stroke the skin around his genitals, but leave his penis and scrotum out for a while. Touch them fleetingly, as if by accident, with the back of your hand. Then let your lips join your hands, still avoiding his best parts. Get nearer and nearer to his genitals, then start to touch and kiss him there, shyly at first. Kiss the tip of his penis until he's going mad, and then allow him to slowly come in all the way. Repeat this delicate torture a few times, before you finally give in to his need.

Foreplay Favourites

The results of the multi-choice survey show that in Ireland passionate kisses are a clear winner when it comes to good foreplay.

What couples do during foreplay

Passionate Kisses	82%
Caressing the Genitals	76%
Caressing the Breasts	73%
Oral Kisses	64%
Teasing All Over	61%

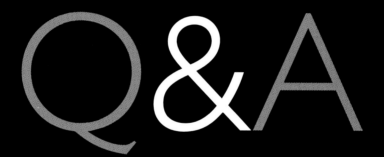

Whenever my husband is ready for sex, he expects me to be ready as well. He pinches my nipples for a minute, gives me a quick rub between the legs and that's it. What can I do about this?

Your husband has to understand that a woman doesn't get all excited by the push of a button. While men often manage to respond almost instantly to sexual stimulation, women take much longer to get aroused. This is a biological fact that has been proved in innumerable surveys and experiments. Tell your husband that you need more foreplay to get into the right mood. A quick rub between the legs won't do the trick. He needs to stimulate you properly before he advances any further. If he doesn't know how to do it, show him.

How long does it take for a woman to be ready for sex? I want to make sure to give my girlfriend enough foreplay.

On average, it takes between 20 and 30 minutes until a woman is ready for sex, but there are huge deviations in both directions. While some women are more than happy with 15 minutes, others need an hour. To find out how long your girlfriend loves to have foreplay, just keep teasing and caressing her until she takes the initiative to go further herself.

How can I tell whether she has had enough foreplay and is physically ready for sex?

Try the finger test – check with the tip of your finger whether your lover's vaginal entrance is moist enough.

My husband touches me during foreplay but never gets it right. I'm too shy to tell or show him how I like being caressed and I could never touch myself while I'm with him. What else can I do?

If you are too shy to talk about your sexual needs and preferences, you have to take the initiative in another way. During foreplay, get on top of your husband. Sit on him to rub yourself off his penis. You can try this discreetly to see how your partner reacts, but I'm sure that he'll enjoy it, especially when he sees how it turns you on.

I have never had sex yet. I came close on a few occasions, but then backed off because I was worried of getting pregnant. Then I was ready to go ahead, but my vagina was too dry to allow intercourse. What could be the reason?

In most cases a dry vagina is a sign of a lack of sexual arousal. Your fear of getting pregnant probably contributes to the problem. To make sure that your vagina gets moist enough for intercourse, use contraceptives to protect yourself against unwanted pregnancy. Then take enough time for foreplay. Don't try to have intercourse before your body is ready for it.

We have a long foreplay, and I do my best to make my wife come when we sleep together but sometimes I would love to just take her. All the caressing and rubbing she needs to climax sort of spoils sex for me. It would be great to have sex the way I love it myself at least from time to time

That's fair enough. If you normally play it her way, I'm sure your partner won't mind you having it your own way once in a while. Most women actually love to just be taken the odd time. To make sure your wife isn't disappointed or even annoyed, explain to her beforehand what you are up to, and ask her whether it's alright to just take her. I'm sure she won't refuse your wish but will be as excited about it as yourself.

I like to have my nipples kissed and nibbled during foreplay but my husband doesn't show much interest in my breasts. He prefers to touch and kiss my bum, my belly and the insides of my legs, where I don't feel much. I am afraid he might get angry when I tell him. After all, he always spends a lot of time with foreplay to please me.

There is no point in having a long foreplay if it doesn't arouse you. Next time your husband is kissing your belly, move his head up to your breasts. I'm sure he'll get the idea. Tell or show him how much you like it. He will be more than happy to find out what really turns you on.

What can I do about my wife's inhibitions? In bed she presses her legs together so firmly that I have to force my hand into the right place to begin foreplay.

Obviously your wife isn't too pleased by the sex she is getting. When she presses her legs together, don't force your hand in. Try a less direct approach. After all, foreplay doesn't start with rubbing the clitoris. Take your wife into your arms, have a cuddle, share a deep kiss, caress her back and shoulders. You might be ready for sex within no time, but please take into account that women need much longer than men to get into the right mood.

I love a good cuddle, lots of kisses and tenderness before making love. My husband is not into that at all. In bed, he more or less just jumps on me. When I complain, he says he doesn't need any foreplay, and that it's only a waste of time. What can I do to make him more understanding of my needs?

Tell your husband how you feel. He has to realise how much you miss tenderness in your relationship. Your husband might not need much foreplay, but he has to grant you that extra bit of time to make you happy in bed.

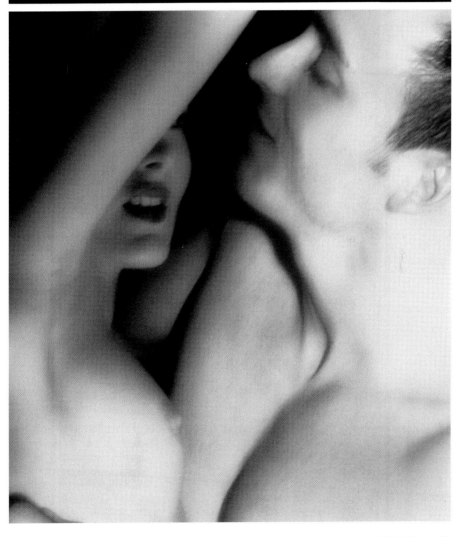

7 Location! Location!

Sex Around the House

Reading the next few pages will make you look around other folks' homes in a different way, and with a good bit of curiosity.

Sitting on their couch, you'll be thinking that they've most likely made love on it, now and then. Seeing their bathtub or shower stall, you'll wonder how they would fit into that together. Having dinner with friends at their kitchen table, you'll wonder whether they've had sex on it.

'When we have the house to ourselves, we do it all over the place,' admits Sheila (41). 'When we moved in we promised each other to make love everywhere. And we have kept that promise. The only place where we didn't make love yet is the loo. We tried — but due to a laughing fit we failed.'

Couples don't need to restrict their lovemaking to the bedroom. There are so many other exciting spots for them to explore. Two out of every three Irish people (65%) have had sex on the couch, almost as many (62%) have tried it on the floor. Four out of ten (42%) have made love in the shower or bathtub. On chairs and tables, leaning against the fireplace or sitting on a vibrating washing machine, are also popular. Irish people are doing it everywhere.

There is hardly a place around the house that has not being used for sexual frolics. The washing machine is appreciated for its vibrations, the fireplace for its soothing crackle and the cupboard under the stairs for just being ridiculous. One of the hottest places is the windowsill. Turn off the lights, so nobody can gaze in at you, then make love leaning against the windowsill, both of you gazing out into the night sky.

Let's have a closer look at the hot spots around the house.

Couch

'The first time I ever had sex on a couch was when I was 17 and still living with my parents', remembers Maureen (26). 'I was dating Brian, my husband now. My parents were out for the night and we had the house to ourselves. After lots of kisses and some heavy petting, we just got carried away – we had our first time right then and there, on the couch in my parents' sitting room. My folks would have thrown a fit if they had caught us.'

Not only young couples get carried away on the cosy couch. Two thirds of us have had the same experience. When you are cuddling on the couch at night, listening to romantic music or watching a movie, it's so inviting you'll want to make love right there and then instead of bothering to go to bed. After all, you don't want to spoil the mood.

Floor

Six out of ten (62%) have made love on the floor. Some go for the freezing kitchen or bathroom tiles, while most prefer a soft rug or carpet. In front of the fireplace is the favourite spot. Experienced fans of sex on the floor choose a position that avoids continuous rubbing of knees or elbows against the carpet, as this leaves burn-like abrasions on your skin.

'I call them carpet burns', grins Sven (31). 'As much as I try to avoid them, in the end I get carried away and suffer them anyway. So my pals at the running club are always up to date on my love life, as it's impossible to hide these abrasions. And nobody believes me anymore when I tell them I just took an unfortunate fall.'

Shower and Bathtub

Sex in the water is one of our favourite sexual dreams. And for most of us it is much more than a mere dream – we actually go ahead and try it out. Four out of ten Irish couples have enjoyed sex in the shower or bathtub. It's not easy to practice, but it's definitely worth a try.

The dream position under the shower is him lifting her up to sit on his penis, while she encircles his neck with her arms and his thighs with her legs. Only try this out if both of you have something solid to hang on to, just in case you lose your balance. Try out a safer option first: he lifts up one of her legs to have it rest on his hip while she clings to his body. If that doesn't work, he can sit down in the shower stall, with her sitting or kneeling on his lap. It's not that adventurous but you will still get a special kick from the water pouring all over you.

And let's not forget oral sex – try out the old game of soaping each other off, and then checking out whether you have done a thorough job.

'Whenever I soap off my husband's penis, he insists that I taste him afterwards to make sure he's clean enough,' Sonya (32) admits. 'Sometimes I think that the only reason he ever gets me into the shower for is to scrub him off, and then have me check whether he tastes good enough.'

Chair

One out of three Irish couples have had sex on a chair. This kinky adventure is normally planned. You don't just get carried away while you're sharing a chair with your loved one. It is more like a crazy idea that pops into your mind and won't let go.

This is the best position: while he sits down on the chair, she sits on his lap, facing him. With her feet on the ground, she can move upon his penis at her own pace, pinning him down with the weight of her body. If the chair is solid, she can risk moving her legs up to rest them over his shoulders.

'Sex on a chair is even better if you don't face your guy, but turn your back to him,' explains Liz (26). 'You can change the angle of penetration by leaning back into him, sitting straight upon him, or moving your body forwards. If you have something solid in front of you to hold on to, you can even lift your feet off the ground to more or less lie on his lap.'

Kitchen Table

Millions of kitchen tables are used for much more than china and cutlery. They become scenes of erotic adventures. Normally it's not more than a quickie that takes place: she leans over the table while he takes her from behind. Or, if the table is solid and can take a good bit of rocking, she sits on the table's edge while he stands in front of her.

So next time you are over at your friends' for dinner, think about what else might get served at their table. And whenever you get a new kitchen table and chairs for yourself, test how solid they are before you buy them. You never know, it might come in handy one day.

Our Favorite Sex Spots – Around the House

Couch	65%
Floor	62%
Shower/bathtub	42%
Chair	35%
Kitchen table	19%
Fireplace	13%
Washing machine	8%

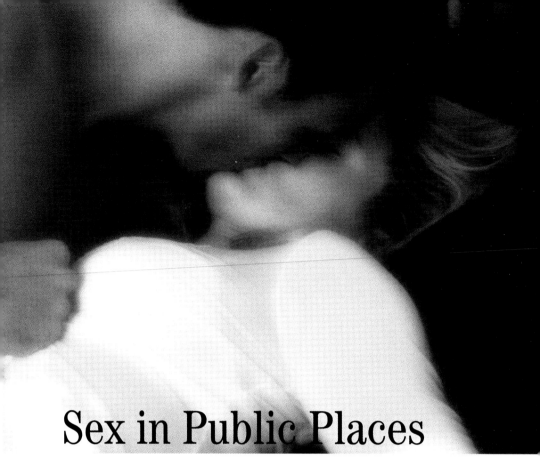

Sex in Public Places

Two thirds of Irish people (66%) have had sex in a car. Looking at a crowd, it's hard to work out who these folks might be. Some look so serious that you can't imagine them doing anything out of the ordinary. Others look like they never have any sex at all. But still two out of every three have had a go at it in a car – hard to believe but true.

Laura (54) falls into that category. With her meticulously coiffed hair and Queen of England style hat and handbag, you couldn't in your wildest dreams imagine her making out on the back seat of a car, but she does exactly that when she feels up to it.

'When my husband and I come home from the pub on a Friday night, we stop in this small alleyway before we drive home to our children. Sometimes you just have to do something naughty.'

There are many other places where you could stumble across a couple making out anytime, like the pub, your workplace, or a dark staircase in your apartment block.

Car

The inner life of a car can be amazing, especially when the wheels are parked behind the pub, in public parking places, or in a semi-discreet lover's lane. Steamed up windows and squeaking shock absorbers are almost sure signs of an erotic interior.

Not only youngsters, with nowhere else to go, make out in the car. Couples with a perfectly private and comfortable bedroom enjoy having sex in their wheels as well.

The sex games taking place in cars range from mutual masturbation and oral sex to sexual intercourse.

'My wife read somewhere that guys are mad about having sex in their car,' grins Tom (51). 'So after almost 30 years of marriage she attacked me in the car one night, following a tip she got on how to spice up your sex life. It completely took me by surprise, but we ended up making passionate love on the passenger seat. And our car has seen much more action since.'

Disco/Night-club

Almost one out of every three Irish people (31%) has had sex at a disco or a night-club and the figures are rising. Hot spots to make out in at the disco are the toilets and the movie rooms.

'Most of our guests leave their normal self with all its inhibitions behind when they step over our threshold,' explains barman Brian (27). 'They are completely different people in here. Last weekend I caught a couple hiding in the corner, leaning against the back of one of our powerful bass loudspeakers to catch the vibes. The guy had his pants down on his ankles. What could I do? I looked the other way, as did everybody else who must have seen them. Once both parties are happy and no harm is being done, I don't have a problem.'

Workplace

It is an entertaining thought to imagine your colleagues, or even your boss, making passionate love somewhere on the premises during working hours. A red 'do not disturb' light gets another meaning if you think about it like that. More than one out of six Irish people (19%) has done it: a quickie leaning over the writing desk or sitting on the office chair, a few minutes of passion in an old storeroom or in a company van in the parking lot.

'With all those modern open plan offices it's getting more and more difficult to find a private space for a few minutes', complains Melanie (46). 'I have had an affair with my boss for more than eight years, but since our offices got modernised, there is no privacy anymore. The only safe place left to us is an old and forgotten storage room, but it will have to do. You know the old saying, "Where there's a will, there's a way."'

Pub

It's hard to imagine, but even the pub isn't left out, one out of six Irish men and women (18%) have had sex in the pub. The main sex spots are the toilets, followed by the backyard.

'We once got all the empty barrels rolling,' remembers Dylan (22). 'They were piled up neatly, but we were having a quickie leaning against them. I had to run off with my pants around my ankles not to get caught. My then girlfriend never forgave me – I left her behind in the mess, while she was frantically grabbing bits and pieces of her clothing.'

School/College

Schools and colleges are places with a vibrant sex life. One out of four Irish students meets a sexual partner at school or college, and one out of seven (15%) actually makes love on the school grounds or the college campus. Favourite places are the sports hall, shower rooms and deserted classrooms.

Others

One of the strangest sex spots is a staircase. Most staircases are cold and uncomfortable, with no visible erotic appeal whatsoever, except the danger that you might get caught at any time. In an elevator, at least the sensation of moving is added to the excitement. But then, it's not easy to find elevators everywhere, while staircases are waiting to be explored wherever you go.

'I have given up on elevators,' says Eddie (38). 'I have tried so many times to have a quickie with my girlfriend, but we always got interrupted before I could even get my penis in.'

An interesting trend shows that more and more sex takes place in fitness centres.

'I am not astonished by that,' explains George (29). 'Most of our regulars are in great shape, and more and more of them, especially the women, dress sexy. It is no wonder when they put on a bit of extra steam in the mixed sauna.'

Our Favorite Sex Spots – In Public Places

Car	66%
Disco/Night-club	31%
Workplace	19%
Pub	18%
Staircase	17%
School/College	15%
Fitness centre	5%
Elevator	4%
Cinema	3%

Sex Outdoors

If you have never tried it – give sex outdoors a chance. It is a great way to spice up your sex life. The most appealing aspect about sex in the open is the natural environment, the fresh air and the background noises, like breaking waves, rustling grass or humming bees. And of course there's the danger of being caught, which mysteriously adds to the excitement, unveiling people's exhibitionistic streak.

If you are too shy to try it at home, go away for a weekend, or try it on your next holidays.

'I love to have sex on the beach, in bright daylight, and among people. They have to be far enough away not to be able to call over, but near enough to realise what must be going on. I just sit on my guy's lap or lie down on his belly, with my bikini still on. Then we make love in slow languid movements so it's not too obvious. Sybil (24)

'I once made out with a girl in a meadow. We didn't scout out the place, just put my jacket down, a couple of cans of beer, and some sandwiches. We quickly forgot about our picnic, and got busy making love. Afterwards we must have dozed for a couple of minutes when suddenly I felt something woolly scraping against my leg. It was a sheep having the leftovers of our picnic!' Brian (26)

There are basically two sides to having sex outdoors: one is the overwhelming romanticism of rolling waves and rosy sunsets, the other is the nuisance of ants in your pants and sand all over your skin. The romantic aspect clearly beats the bad points and makes us try to ignore these little nuisances. In Ireland our favourite place for sex outdoors is in the park. One out of three Irish people have tried it out and most of them more than once.

'There are spots in our park where you can make love for hours on end without anybody disturbing you. You can see the odd runner in the distance, and the deer might come over to have a peek, but otherwise it's just my girlfriend and me in the high grass. But I have to admit that the

fact that you might be seen by others anytime, gives outdoor sex an extra thrill.' Paul (33)

The beach is Ireland's second favourite spot. One out of four Irish people (25%) have made love on the beach.

'There is nothing like it,' remembers Catherine (19). 'Lying under palm trees on the soft sand, and the man of your dreams making love to you.'

Lovebirds often frequent fields and alleyways as well. Balconies and backyards are also favourite love locations. Peeping into your neighbours' backyard on a mild summer's night, you might well get an unexpected glimpse of their love life.

Park

One out of every three men and women in Ireland (36%) has had sex in the park. The favourite spot is at the root of a huge, sheltering tree, closely followed by nestling into a patch of high grass. The high grass makes you invisible as long as you keep your head, and the rest of your body, down. Rustling around you, the grass blades' soothing whisper helps you to forget about the rest of the world.

'All summer we had this crazy idea of making love in the high grass,' admits Kevin (36). 'It was August when one night we finally set out with a blanket and a bottle of wine. For once, my girlfriend wanted to be on top, to be on the lookout. While she was moving on my hips, she glanced around to make sure that nobody was sneaking in on us. We repeated this several times since, as it was just fantastic.'

Beach

Making love on the beach is a special treat, day and night. In the daytime, the sun on your skin increases the flow of your hormones and your lust for your lover while at night, the sound of the waves and the starry sky above make you long for a bit of romance. If you are new to the game it's best to choose a spot on the beach near other couples. Normally each lovers' nest is respected by other couples. People might stroll over for a discreet glimpse but they won't disturb you.

On a tropical island, the best place to make love is at the water's edge. Let the surf caress you, while your bodies find a rhythm in sync with the waves. In the Mediterranean the perfect spot is under a palm tree, while in colder climate it's better to seek the shelter of the dunes.

Field

Making love in a field is not for the faint-hearted. You are surrounded by the strangest cacophony of noises: rustling, cracking, squeaking – whatever you can imagine. This is bad enough during the day, but can be really scary at night. Bringing a flashlight doesn't help. On the contrary, in its long shadows you're never sure what you might see or what might come creeping towards you. But then in this part of the world it's not tigers or lions creeping up on you that you have to worry about. You just need to watch out for a harmless horse or cow. So try it out. If you want to go for it at night, cuddle up in a cosy sleeping bag for comfort.

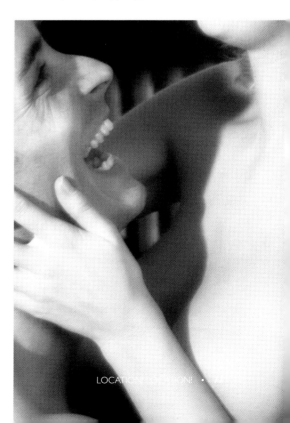

Balcony or Backyard

Outdoors, but still at home – this is the ideal starter pack for outdoor-sex-enthusiasts. A private backyard can't be beaten. Comfortable garden furniture, especially padded sun beds, can be used for much more than sunbathing and barbecues. Lovemaking in the backyard is seldom seen in daylight. To make sure that they are not going to be spotted by nosy neighbours, most couples wait until it gets dark.

'We often stretch out on a sunbed in our pavilion after dark,' tells Mike (33). 'With the gas burner on, it's cosy even if there is a drizzle. Sharing a glass of wine, we talk and snuggle half of the night. I can't wait for our neighbours to go to bed, for only then my wife allows me to undress her and make love to her.'

Alleyway

One out of seven Irish people has had sex in a quiet and dark alleyway. Most couples who end up in an alley simply have nowhere else to go. Apart from drunken couplings and one-night stands between strangers there is a good bit of prostitution going on in the dark shadows and corners of Ireland's alleyways as well. It's a place where you need to have your wits about you – so be careful.

Others

A romantic scene for lovers that has seen better times is the hayloft: only 20 years ago, it still was a popular spot for making out.

'We used to roll in the hay before we got married,' remembers Vera (45). 'I loved the smell of the fresh hay, but that stuff stuck all over you when you were finished, giving away what you've been up to. It felt great anyway.'

Meadows and forests are loosing out as well. But then, there's not so many around anymore anyway.

Our Favorite Sex Spots – Outdoors	
Park	36%
Beach	25%
Field	24%
Alleyway	16%
Balcony or backyard	13%
Hayloft	4%

Q&A

I went to the park with my girlfriend to make love, but she couldn't find a spot where the grass was high enough for her taste. Since then the desire for making love in the grass hasn't left my mind. How can I persuade my girlfriend to play along?

Tell her how much this fantasy turns you on. It's only natural that she's a bit shy about having sex in the open. So go to the park on your own to scout out the right spot. Before you bring her out there, make sure she's in the right mood for this adventure.

With my last boyfriend I enjoyed sex in unusual places, in the sauna of our gym, a storage room at our workplace, out in the park, even on a train one night. The guy I'm going out with now is terribly boring in comparison. I've been trying hard to seduce him in public places, but he says he couldn't stand the embarrassment of getting caught.

As much as I can understand your hunger for adventure, your guy's worries are understandable as well. Being caught with your pants around your ankles is just not everybody's idea of having fun. In the worst case scenario, it can even get you into legal trouble. That doesn't mean you have to do without it. Try to show your boyfriend slowly but surely how exciting sexual adventures can be. Seduce him in unusual places where it is highly unlikely that anybody could surprise you. Once he gets used to that, you can try to take things a bit further.

On our next holidays, I want to make love to my wife on the beach, but I'm afraid she might rebuff me like she always does when I suggest something out of the ordinary. Is there a way I could bring her to fulfil my wish this one time?

On holidays your chances are definitely much better than at home. Don't be too bold about your plan – that would probably frighten your wife off from the start. Instead, try to get her used to the idea step by step. On the first night, take her to the beach for a walk and a few kisses. Next night, go a bit further, and so on. Be loving and romantic. It needs a lot of patience, but you have a good chance to get your erotic dream fulfilled at last.

When my wife prepares dinner, I love to embrace her from behind and rub my penis against her bum. Although she says she likes that, she always pushes me off after a while. I would love to take her right there in the kitchen.

That sounds like a good idea. Be a bit more insistent. Tell your wife how much you would like to make love to her in the kitchen. Nibble her neck, whisper endearments into her ear, and play with her breasts while you embrace her. To make sure she can't refuse because of some lame excuse, you could try closing the curtains and locking the doors before you playfully attack her.

What would be a good position to seduce him in the kitchen?

You could seduce him at the table after dinner, dressed up in a mini, secretly wearing nothing underneath. After a bit of teasing, place your legs right and left of the chair, and then slowly sit down, with your back turned towards him. I'm sure he'll go mad when he sees your mini slipping up, as you lower yourself onto his lap.

How can my boyfriend and I make love in the bathtub?

While he lies back, you can kneel above him. Or, to make it more comfortable for you, he can kneel at one end of the tub, while you stretch out at the other end, with your legs resting on the rim of the tub. He then has to place his hands around your buttocks to move you towards him.

How can we have sex in the shower? I am more than a foot taller than my wife, so we can't do it standing up.

If you have strong arms, and your wife is light enough, lift her up to sit on your forearms, encircling your thighs with her legs, and with her arms wrapped around your neck. Holding her bum in your hands, you can move her up and down to make love. Please be careful when you try this position. Make sure there's an anti-slip shower mat, and that there's something solid to hold on to in case you lose your balance.

Is it safe to make love in the water? Will the water get trapped inside, or does it run out again?

Making love in the water is harmless. Even when you only go for a swim, or soak in your bathtub, water can get into your vagina, but it simply runs out again later.

I would love to have sex in the shower. I've done it a few times with my former boyfriend, and it was the best sex I've ever had. How can I make my fiancé play along? Should I tell him about my experience, or keep quiet and try to coax him around?

It's never a good idea to confront a guy with your past sexual experiences, especially when they've been fantastic. Just tell your fiancé that you'd love to slip into the shower with him, without mentioning sex. Then soap him off, start with his back, then slowly work your way around to his genitals. I'm sure you'll manage to get him into the right mood for more. Make sure there's an anti-slip shower mat in place, in case your wish gets fulfilled.

My girlfriend and I both want to sleep together for the first time. The problem is that she doesn't want sex in my car, but that's the only place where we could have it. Isn't making love in the car much better than not having sex at all? I don't want to wait any longer.

Don't spoil things with your impatience. It's only normal that your girlfriend wants your first time to be perfect. While sex in the car can be great fun, it just doesn't fit into a girl's dreams of romance and tenderness. Wait until you come up with a better idea. You can enjoy your first time much more in the right surroundings.

I would love to try sex in public places, but I always back down at the last moment being too shy. What can I do to overcome my shyness?

Go away for a weekend to fulfill your dream. It is much easier to overcome your shyness when you are in a place where nobody knows you. Scout out a perfect location in daytime, then go back in the evening. Start with kissing and touching, taking your time to progress further. Even if people see you, you will notice that most of them don't care what you're doing, they will leave you alone and keep their distance. It's only a very few who would be bold enough to come closer to watch or even confront you. Once you have realised that, you should be able to shed your shyness and make love.

My husband always sneaks up on me in the kitchen, whispering sexy things, trying to seduce me. I always make him stop, although part of me wants him to go all the way. I'm just too shy to have sex in the kitchen, or anywhere else in the house. What could we do in the kitchen anyway?

You can have lots of erotic fun in the kitchen. So try to overcome your shyness, and let your husband have his way; I'm sure he's worked out the best position in his fantasy.

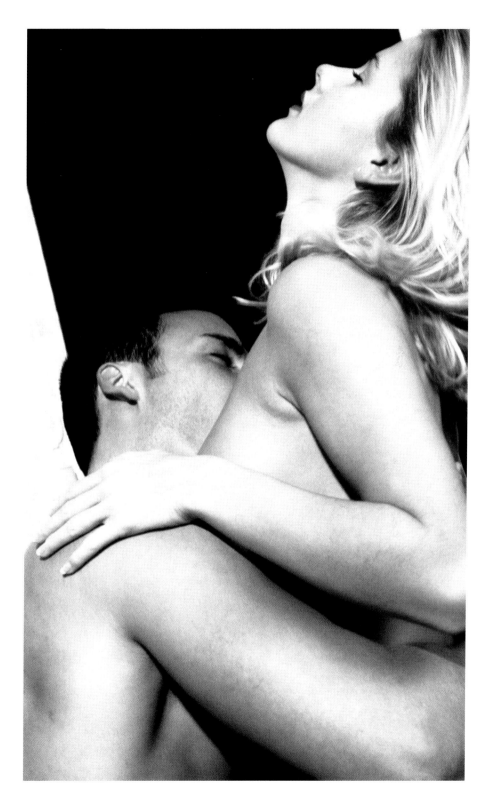

8 Positions

Favourite Sex Positions

When it comes to the choice of sex positions all around the globe there isn't much harmony in people's beds.

The general attitude is that it is much nicer to let your partner take over the more active role, while you enjoy lovemaking from a lazy, more passive position.

In Ireland nearly three quarters of all Irish women between 16 and 40 (73%) want their lover to play the leading role in the bedroom, while only one quarter (27%) prefer to be in charge themselves. The answer isn't very different when you ask men about their wishes. Nearly two thirds of them (62%) want their women to play the active and more dominant part while only one third (38%) wants to hold the reins themselves. The best way to make sure your partner takes command is to get them on top when you make love.

'This is a constant fight between my husband and myself,' explains Margaret (41) from Co. Dublin. 'We both want the other one to get on top to spoil us, while we lie back and lazily enjoy the pleasures. We normally agree on a compromise. First, I sit on top of him to let him live out his fantasy. Shortly before he comes, we change positions because I can't climax without feeling his weight upon my body.'

It is not only laziness that makes people prefer it if their partner plays the more active role. Many people find it a big turn on to be 'taken' and to give in to their lover's desires. And then there is always the chance that your partner might try out something new that he or she has heard of, read or merely fantasised about.

'That is the main reason why I want my lover to dominate our lovemaking,' explains Roy (23) from Co. Westmeath. 'I know this is unusual, but she is so full of new ideas that I feel like I'm the luckiest man on earth. My lovemaking is lame and boring compared to hers. The only problem is that she wants me to take the initiative most of the time. That puts me under immense pressure to act up to her expectations.'

A list of Irish people's favourite sex positions highlights men and women's mutual desire to be dominated. While women vote for the missionary position, Irish men prefer their woman to be on top. Second in the women's hit list is woman on top, while the men voted for 'from behind'. Women love sex from behind as well, but most find it difficult to come that way. That sounds like bad news for all the guys who'd love to take their women doggy style, but it's not that bad at all. Just caress your lover's clitoris with your hand while you make love to her in this position – that should do the trick. So it's up to you to make her come and encourage her to enjoy sex from behind. If you succeed in giving her this pleasure, she'll change her attitude for sure and will want to make love this way more often.

Almost one in three Irish women and one in four men count the side position as one of their favourites.

'It is nice for a change but I wouldn't want to try it every time we make love,' comments Deirdre (37) from Co. Dublin. 'It's not easy in a technical way. First of all, it is very awkward to get him in, and then he easily slips out again. The positive aspect is that I can touch myself while my partner makes love to me lying behind me on his side.'

The standing and sitting positions or a combination of both are growing in popularity. Inspired not only by their fantasies, but by more and more explicit love scenes in films as well, many young couples experiment with unusual and even awkward positions.

'I first saw this great position in a film and then had to try it out myself. This guy held a woman on his forearms, while she wrapped her legs around his waist. He moved her upon him, while he was gazing into her eyes. Unfortunately, my boyfriend and I didn't manage to replay this scene, but at least we came near it, with me sitting on the edge of a table, while my boyfriend stood in front of me.' Jane (23) from Co. Cavan.

Ireland's Top Six Sex Positions

WOMEN	TOTAL
Man on top	66%
Woman on top	59%
From behind	41%
Side position	32%
Sitting	19%
Standing	16%

MEN	TOTAL
Woman on top	62%
From behind	52%
Man on top	43%
Side position	25%
Standing	21%
Sitting	19%

What is Most Important in a Sex Position?

The most important aspect of a sex position for both men and women is that they can feel their partner intensely. Women want to be able to achieve an orgasm easily, while men are more interested in being able to hold their orgasm back as long as possible. For 44% of women and 36% of men it's a big turn on to be able to watch their partner's face while they make love to them. This way they can not only look at their beloved's features but they also get to witness their lust and desire.

'To watch my woman come is the best moment for me,' explains Kevin (31) from Co. Sligo. 'To first see the ecstasy in her expression and then the happy afterglow of her orgasm.'

'What are the most important factors in a sex position?'

WOMEN	TOTAL
That I can feel my partner intensely	74%
That I achieve an orgasm easily	59%
That I can watch my partner's face	44%
That no acrobatics are involved	46%
That the climax can be delayed as long as possible	28%

MEN	TOTAL
That I can feel my partner intensely	73%
That I achieve an orgasm easily	34%
That I can watch my partner's face	36%
That no acrobatics are involved	25%
That the climax can be delayed as long as possible	51%

Experimenting

Experimenting in bed is becoming more and more popular. An astonishing 72% of Irish women and 84% of men like to try out new positions from time to time. Most get their inspiration from magazines and films, followed by erotic literature. Wherever the ideas come from – lovers want to give them a go.

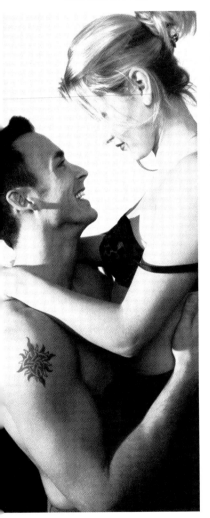

Couples have started to talk openly about new positions. That doesn't mean that all their sexual dreams are being fulfilled, but at least they are being discussed, and the best ones have a chance of becoming a reality. The growing will to experiment doesn't stop at the bedroom door either: 73% of women and 84% of men like positions that would allow them to have spontaneous sex in unusual places.

'I love to experiment with standing up positions,' grins Orla (27) from Co. Dublin. 'You can do it practically everywhere, in an alleyway, in the park leaning against a tree. We have even done it on the staircase of our apartment block. I prefer face-to-face positions, and try out new variations all the time.'

While most women are willing enough to talk about experimenting, they are still more reluctant than men to actually go ahead and try something new, especially the more advanced and elaborate experiments, like trying out several positions in one session. This is a concern many women share. As Sabrina (26) from Co. Wicklow explains:

'It's fun to try out something new, but I feel a bit like a laboratory rat when a guy expects me to work with him through a whole catalogue of new positions that he has on his mind. When I try out something new and don't like it, I want to go back to something familiar to make sure I don't get completely frustrated.'

The Old Favourites

Although the will to give new ideas a try is clearly increasing, Irish men on average still know only 12 different sex positions, while Irish women on average can't think of more than eight.

So let's look at some old favourites and some new exciting positions to give their sexual fantasies a little boost.

1 Man on Top *You all know the legendary missionary position: she lies on her back with her legs opened and her knees pulled up at a slight angle while he lies on top of her between her legs, supporting his weight on his arms. This classic position is, of course, not the only way to make love with the man on top.*

Instead of spreading her legs, the woman can keep them closed or even slightly cross them at the ankles. This way the vagina feels much tighter, adding extra pleasure. He can't get in deep, but the effect of tightness more than makes up for that. Also, there is a good chance that his penis will rub against her clitoris with every movement, especially if he doesn't rest his weight on his arms, but mainly upon her body, with his arms encircling her shoulders.

In another variation, she encircles her legs around his hips with her ankles crossing over his bum, and then hugs him close with a squeeze. The higher the legs are raised the deeper the penetration. Better still, she moves her legs up and over his shoulders. It sounds a bit awkward, but this position is hard to beat, as it allows the deepest penetration ever. If his penis is too big for this position, encircle its shaft with your hand to keep him from getting in too deep.

'My guy absolutely loves this position. The first time I brought my legs up and wrapped them around his neck, he went absolutely mad with desire, he hadn't experienced anything like that ever before. He ran his hands up and down my legs, while his penis went mad between them.' Carol (24) from Co. Cork.

2 Woman on Top *In the standard version of the position 'woman on top', the man basically has to do nothing but lie back while the woman kneels over him, sitting on his crotch. It is not easy to get your bits together this way, especially if the man's erection is so firm that it's leaning against his belly. Just give him a helping hand to guide him in. Once you have managed that, it is mainly up to you to control the depth and rhythm of penetration. To take him in as deep as possible, arch your spine back and rest your hands either on his upper legs or on the bed beside them. For increased closeness, move* your upper body down to lie upon his chest while your pelvis keeps moving rhythmically on his hips.

Another good tip is to lie down on him with your legs stretched out flat. With her thighs closed, a woman feels much tighter and that's a guarantee for extra pleasure.

And then this technique is sure to give extra pleasure: sit on top of your man, with your back towards his face, leaning your hands onto his legs. Initially this position is a bit tricky, but it promises exquisite ecstasy due to the unusual angle of penetration.

A huge advantage of the woman on top position is the fact that both partners have their hands free to caress and stimulate their lover's as well as their own bodies while they make love.

'Being on top I can control the pace of our lovemaking. I can go fast or slow, teasing him the whole time. I love to see the growing ecstasy on his face.' Maureen (22) from Co. Donegal.

3 From Behind In the
classic doggy-style position, the woman gets down on her hands and knees, while her partner kneels behind her, clutching her hips to move them rhythmically against his crotch. The woman is extremely restricted in her possibilities to actively participate. She can stretch out a hand to caress his testicles, touch his anus or touch herself, but that's about it.

'My absolute favourite is to take her from behind. She kneels on the bed in front of me with her buttocks turned up to meet me. I either grab her hips with both my hands to move them against me or I use my hands to play with her breasts.'Martin (35) from Co. Waterford.

Sex from behind allows extra deep penetration, so it's ideal for men with a shorter than average-sized penis. From medium-sized onwards, he tends to get in too deep. In that case, it helps to encircle the base of his penis shaft with a restricting hand.

'My lad's penis is barely five inches long when erect, and he is very conscious about it. But when we make love from behind, I have to encircle the base of his penis with my thumb and forefinger, otherwise he gets in too deep.' Elaine (21) from Co. Dublin.

While a majority of Irish men love doggy-style, women often feel uncomfortable and exposed in this position, with their rear end sticking up invitingly. It helps to lie down flat on your belly, even though your guy's weight is then on your back which can mean that you are smothered by pillows and mattress. As long as this doesn't bother you this position feels great, especially as it allows your man to stimulate your clitoris while you make love. When you lie down flat on your belly, it's almost impossible for his penis to slip in. To make entrance easier, place a cushion under your hips to make the angle of penetration less awkward. Once he is in, you can spread your legs, stretch them out or clutch them together to vary the sensation.

The same goes for him. He can kneel over his lover or lie on top of her. If he lies upon her, he can enclose her legs with his own, stretch his legs out to rest upon hers or can clutch them together to lie between her thighs. There are so many variations of this position that you could easily spend a good few nights experimenting.

4 Side Position

Also known as spooning, side positions are a great way of increasing the feeling of intimacy between two partners. They are meant for patient souls who like to prolong their lovemaking, as most side positions don't invite fast movements and don't allow deep penetration.

You can lie belly to belly, facing each other. This way your hands are free to caress your partner's body. You can both keep your legs stretched out flat or move one leg up to encircle your partner's leg or thigh.

In another variation he cuddles up behind her and then encircles her in his arms. To make entry easier, she can pull a leg back over his hip to let it rest behind his bum.

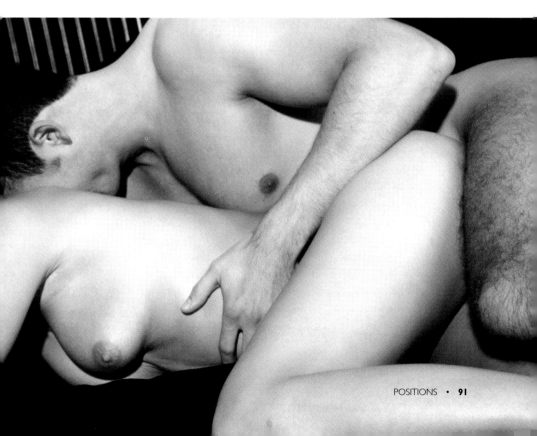

If she needs much longer than him to get an orgasm, here is the ideal position: with your man lying on his side facing towards you, move both your legs over your man's hips. Stay half-lying on your back, half on your side in order to clutch him. In this position, both of you have a hand free to caress her clitoris while all other movement comes to an almost complete standstill. He has to hold still to delay his own orgasm. Even then, she can still feel his penis pulsing impatiently in her vagina. Shortly before she is about to climax, she can start to slightly move her pelvis and so release her partner from the torture of holding still.

5 Sitting The sitting position is a very gentle way to make love. The most well-known variation is the man sitting upright on the bed, with his legs stretched out at a slight angle, while the woman sits on top of him, facing him, encircling her legs behind his back. It is not easy to make love this way, but it's definitely worth a try. Hold each other tightly while you rock gently back and forward. To make it easier, she can kneel over his lap – but the feeling is not the same!

To change position slightly, lean your bodies backwards to let their weight rest on your elbows or hands. This allows you to move your hips more freely and passionately. As a very sexy, but not easy to manage alternative, she can pull her legs up over his shoulders while either hanging on to him in a close embrace or leaning back to rest her weight on her hands and lower arms. For another change, the man kneels on the bed while the woman sits on his lap. This position is not too popular as his legs tend to fall asleep in the middle of the act. But if they don't it can be very enjoyable.

'This is by far my favourite,' says Ellie (19) from Co. Sligo. 'My boyfriend kneels on the bed and I sit on his lap with my legs folded behind his hips. He holds my bum to keep me in place, and to move me up and down upon him.'

Instead of facing each other, she can sit with her back to him: while he sits on the bed, slightly leaning back, she sits on his lap with her back towards him. You can try the same position with him sitting on a chair instead of on the bed and with her legs pulled up to rest on the chair, while her hands hold onto his legs.

6 Standing The many variations of this position range from the more acrobatic to the stationary. The following classic is quite acrobatic: standing upright, he carries her weight on his forearms, while her arms are wound around his neck and her legs are clasped behind his buttocks. Holding her bum on his hands and forearms, he moves her hips up and down upon his penis. This position is an absolute dream, but it's not easy to carry out. It needs strong arms to hold a woman like that. To make it easier, the man can lean against something, be it a solid table or the hood of a car.

Another classic is the couple standing facing each other. He pulls and holds up one of her legs, then tries to get himself inside, which isn't easy at all, but can be managed with a bit of practice. This is one of the positions that allow you to have sex without bothering too much about undressing. It's best if she's wearing a skirt, which can come in handy when you're in a hurry or find yourself in a spot where you could be seen.

The following is more practical: she stands upright, bent over slightly, while he takes her from behind. Men shouldn't even think about trying this with a tall woman. To come together, she would either have to bend her knees very low, inviting cramps, or he would have to find a crate to step on.

If your girl is taller than you, let her sit on the edge of a low table or any other solid object, while you stand in front of her. Let her encircle your buttocks with her legs to keep you in place or put her legs up to let them rest on your shoulders.

The major advantage of standing positions is undoubtedly that you can practice them practically everywhere. They are ideal for a quickie on a dark staircase, on the beach or a thousand other places – but remember to be careful and don't get caught.

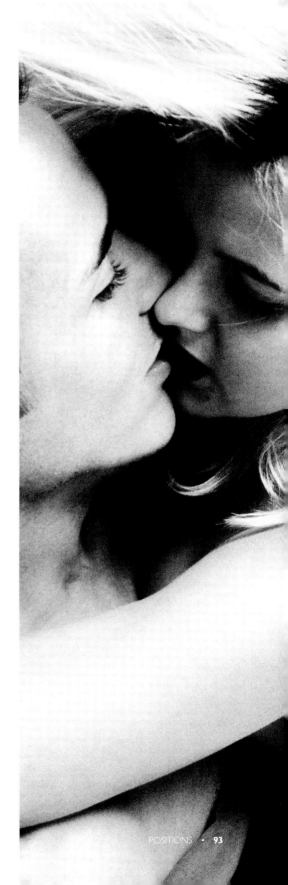

Some New Favourites

Playing Kinky and Checking Out The Kama Sutra

Now let's get away from the standard positions and move on to the more elaborate ones. If you are ever in need of inspiration regarding love techniques and positions, have a look at The Kama Sutra. It is an ancient Sanskrit treatise on the art of love and sexual technique that won't fail to inspire your fantasies.

1 Butterfly Position

In this position, the man stands up while the female lies down on her back in front of him, her legs pointing towards him. She then lifts her pelvis up to meet his penis, with him supporting her. To make love in this position is tricky to say the least, but it's well worth the effort.

2 Rising Position

He kneels on the bed, while she lies on her back facing him with her legs over his shoulders and her pelvis raised to meet his penis. This position allows deep penetration, so give it a try.

3 Chair Position

He lies on his back, with his knees and legs pulled up, like he was providing a chair for his lover to sit on. And that is exactly what she has to do. Facing away from him she takes a seat on his penis. This is such an unusual angle of penetration that it can't fail to arouse.

4 Pressed Position

He kneels on the bed with her lying in front of him on her back with her knees pulled up to her chin, her pelvis raised and the soles of her feet pressing against his chest. As a variation, she can stretch one of her legs out over his shoulder, while her other foot remains pressing against his chest.

5 Lotus Position

She lies on her back with her legs drawn up and folded one over the other like in the famous yoga position, while he kneels upon her. In this position her vagina is pulled up to meet her partner's penis. The only problem is that it is really tough on the woman to hold this position for long.

SEX DICTIONARY

LUST
An extremely strong sexual desire.

KAMA SUTRA
An ancient Indian Sanskrit text on love and sex, above all describing all the sex positions imaginable.

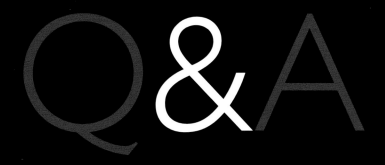

Q&A

I never come when I sleep with my boyfriend but I orgasm easily when I masturbate. Which position allows me best to discreetly touch myself while I sleep with my man?

You can best reach your clitoris when your partner makes love to you from behind, with yourself either kneeling or lying on your side. You can also get on top of him, although in that position it is much more obvious when you start to caress yourself. But then, there is nothing wrong with that especially if it helps you to climax.

My husband wants to try out new positions but I'd rather stick to having him get on top. I am a bit overweight and therefore afraid that I might look ridiculous when we try out something different.

I'm sure that your husband loves you the way you are, so don't be embarrassed to try out new positions. The missionary position isn't necessarily ideal anyway if you have a few extra pounds. Men normally find sex from behind (doggy style) extremely sexy, especially if their woman is the classic curvy type.

I can't make my guy come when I am on top

Try different positions. First, kneel over his lap, so he can watch and touch your breasts while you move upon him. Then lie down on his chest, with your knees still pulled up, and make him clutch your buttocks with his hands to show you the rhythm he likes you to move with. Then stretch out your legs, as this again feels completely different from the other two positions. With a bit of practice you will manage to make him come while you're on top.

He wants me on top all the time. I don't mind getting on top now and then, but I very much prefer my man to play the active role. When I'm on top he just lies back, not even moving his hips, and lets me do all the work.

The problem you describe is a well-known dilemma. Women in general prefer the missionary position, while men want their women to be on top. But of course not every man is as impassive and lazy as yours when he gets his wish fulfilled. So tell your partner why you dislike being on top, then go for a compromise. There is no harm in spoiling him now and then if he agrees to do the same for you in return.

I want to try out the position 'from behind'. But none of the women I've met so far were willing to let me try it. Am I asking too much of them?

Women want to embrace their partner when they make love, especially when they have sex with a new lover for the first time. They feel used when you approach them with exceptional sexual wishes from the very start of your relationship. Okay, sex from behind is not that unusual, but it's still best not to give a woman the impression that it is some special technique of lovemaking you are after.

I don't want to do the missionary position on our first time as my lover might think it's boring. Could you suggest any other positions that are more exciting?

There is nothing wrong with the missionary position – most women prefer it, especially for their first time with a new partner. Much more important than the choice of position is that you show your girlfriend how much you care for her. Spoil her with a long foreplay and keep kissing and caressing her while you make love. Start with the missionary position, and then try to roll over to get her on top.

9 Oral Sex

Erotic kisses are slowly but surely gaining popularity. Our survey shows that one out of every three couples in Ireland love to have oral sex instead of intercourse – they are more than content with intimate kisses for their main menu.

Men have always fancied the special treat of oral sex, while, up to now, women have been much more reluctant. Women are still a bit more reserved than men about giving oral pleasures, and are shyer about receiving them, but the gap between the sexes is closing rapidly.

Women as well as men love oral sex especially as an appetiser during foreplay. Couples enjoy erotic kisses almost everywhere. While women prefer romantic surroundings, men especially love to be spoilt in their car. It is a classic male fantasy to have a woman working away in their lap while they nonchalantly gaze out the window.

'My man is absolutely mad about oral sex when he is driving,' tells Suzanne (22) from Co. Dublin. 'I won't do it; he has to stop somewhere if he wants me to spoil him. I prefer more private surroundings myself.'

To satisfy your partner orally isn't easy. First of all, you need to know the basic technique. And then, even more important, you need to find out which sort of caresses your partner loves most. Let's see which kind of oral kisses and caresses women and men prefer.

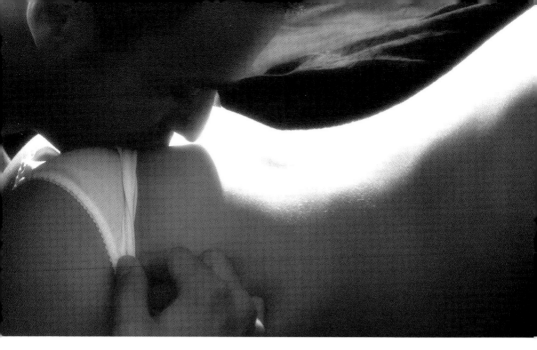

Cunnilingus

Almost two thirds of Irish women (64%) love to feel their clitoris being caressed by their lover's lips and tongue. His lips should nuzzle around her clitoris, while his tongue plays teasingly with her most sensitive spot. The sensation is perfect when he moves his hands caressingly all over her body.

One out of every three Irish women love to feel his tongue inside her vagina, while one out of four likes to get her labia (the lips just outside the vagina) kissed.

Even more important than the right technique is to feel certain that the man likes what he is doing. It is hard for a woman to enjoy something that feels more like a dutiful exercise than an act of lust and love.

So, if your girl calls you 'back up', ask her whether you might stay down for another while. If you enjoy what you are doing, let her know that you love it.

'It is great to just lean back and enjoy his kisses,' explains Catherine (25) from Co. Cork. 'But I need to feel sure that my man enjoys it as well. To make sure, I tease his penis, testicles, and anus while he gives me cunnilingus.'

Fellatio

Two thirds of all Irish men (66%) love to get their penis spoiled by a woman's lips and tongue. For many men it feels best to be in her mouth, while her tongue fools around, teasing him.

Every second guy loves to get his testicles kissed, while only one out of four likes his woman to take them into her mouth – they are just too sensitive, especially in the state of sexual arousal. And women who are usually very careful when they handle a penis, often get carried away when they feel a firm scrotum in their hands or in their mouths. It is just too inviting for them to give it a hearty squeeze.

'I always get nervous when a woman I haven't had sex with yet gets near my testicles,' describes Mike (38) from Co. Galway. 'I have had some really bad experiences. Once there was this woman who took them in her mouth and then started sucking so hard that I thought she was ripping them off. I still get goose bumps when I think about the pain.'

A very special wish, shared by one fourth of all men, is to come in a woman's mouth. The bad news is that women aren't mad about this at all. Their main reservation is still the idea that it is unhygienic. So the best way to introduce a woman to fellatio is to try it in the shower or bathtub, after she has scrubbed you off with her own hands. If she is still reluctant, use a condom. There are fancy ones that taste of banana, strawberry and other delicacies.

Position 69

By far the best and most intimate way to enjoy oral sex is position 69. To receive and give intimate kisses at the same time is about the closest you can ever get to your partner. Almost two out of every three Irish men and women love 'the 69' but it takes a good bit of practice to get comfortable in this position. The numbers 6 and 9 that the position is named after illustrate how your bodies should be arranged. The most common way to practice it is to lie on your side, belly to belly, facing each other, with one of you upside-down. Every couple has to work out their perfect position 69, as it depends not only on personal tastes but on the size and shape of your bodies as well. Once you've managed, it's very rewarding, as you can hardly get any more intimate with your loved one.

'69 is my dream position,' exclaims Ruth (33) from Co. Carlow. 'My husband and I do it so often that we have become experts. Most of the time we even manage to come together. The first few times I wasn't too mad about the taste of his sperm, and spat it out, which was quite unromantic. Now I just swallow it, and it's not bad at all.'

According to our multi-choice survey Irish people think that oral sex is:

WOMEN	TOTAL
The perfect foreplay	48%
Really nice now and then	32%
A must when I have sex	25%
Embarrassing	3%
A torture	3%

MEN	TOTAL
The perfect foreplay	53%
A must when I have sex	28%
Really nice now and then	17%
Embarrassing	5%
A torture	3%

SEX DICTIONARY

CUNNILINGUS
Giving a woman oral sex by licking her clitoris.

DEEP THROAT
Slang term for taking a penis deeply into one's mouth or even down the throat, overcoming the gag reflex.

FELLATIO
Intimately kissing a man's genitals, normally by taking his penis into one's mouth.

POSITION 69
This means mutual oral sex. The number 69 indicates how your bodies have to be positioned – facing each other – to make this work.

GOLDEN RULES

Make sure you are clean when you ask a lover to kiss you intimately.

Moan and groan to show your partner that you appreciate his or her efforts.

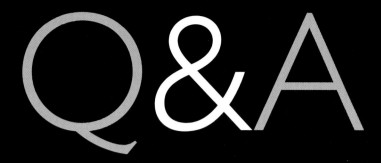

How do you have oral sex with a man? What exactly do you have to do?

To get started, you can kiss and lick your man's penis and testicles. To give him oral sex properly, you take his penis into your mouth and then move your lips up and down it. It's best to hold the base of his penis shaft with your hand to make sure he can't move too vehemently or get in too deep.

Are there any side effects of swallowing his sperm?

Oral sex and swallowing sperm, like other kinds of unprotected sex, can transmit diseases between sexual partners. Otherwise, if both are completely healthy, practising oral sex and swallowing sperm is safe. There are no other side effects, except that you might not like the feel and taste of it.

What is the best position to kiss him orally?

The best way is to kneel between his legs. The penis is most sensitive at its base, and in that position your tongue is perfectly situated to find his most sensitive spots and to give extra pleasure by spoiling his testicles as well.

I keep refusing my husband oral sex, because I don't want him to come in my mouth. What should we do?

Many women share your reservations but that's no reason to reject oral sex altogether. You don't have to make your husband come in your mouth. Spoil him with intimate kisses during foreplay. I'm sure that's a compromise he will be more than happy with.

My lover is so well built that I can't help gagging when giving him oral sex, especially when his movements get faster and he gets in deeper. What can I do to stop gagging?

Don't let him be in charge when you have oral sex. Let him lie down on his back while you sit or lie on top of him. Encircle the base of his penis with your hand to make sure he gets in only as deep as you can manage.

My wife never kisses my penis. She says that I use it to pee, so she wouldn't take it into her mouth. I would be happy enough if she would at least kiss my testicles. With her feeling that way, how can I make her interested in oral sex?

Some women are mad about hygiene. So take a bath before you mention oral sex, and make sure that your wife notices this. To be on the safe side, make her scrub you down herself. After she has washed you, she can hardly refuse to at least caress your testicles with her lips.

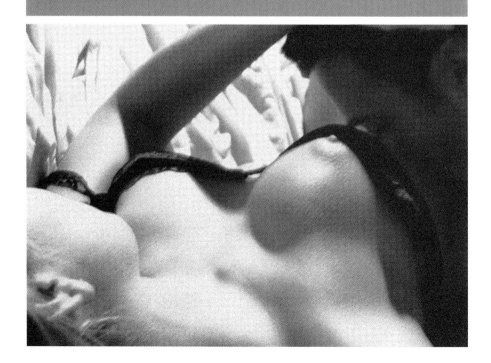

I love to get oral sex, but I can't bring myself
to do the same for my man. I really want to,
but my inhibitions are too strong.

Many of us suffer from inhibitions we were brought up with, one
of them being the myth that genitals are dirty. In ancient times,
when people had a bath once a week, at the most, there might have
been some truth to this, but not nowadays. To feel more
comfortable about kissing your man's penis, take a bath together
and soap him off before you kiss him intimately. If that doesn't do
the trick, use a condom.

Is oral sex safe without a condom?

You can't get pregnant from oral sex, but it is not safe to have
unprotected oral sex due to the risk of STDs. The HIV virus, as
well as other STDs, can be transmitted through cuts, sores, and
mucous membranes (mouth, vagina, anus). The person performing
oral sex is at a much higher risk than the one receiving. I would
strongly recommend that you use a condom, especially with a new
partner.

What are flavoured condoms for? Can I use them for intercourse?

There is indeed a wide range of flavoured condoms, with theoret-
ically the right flavour for every taste, although most fail to fulfil a
gourmet's expectations. Flavoured condoms are mainly used for
oral sex. Sure, you can put them on for intercourse as well, but
what's the point? The vagina doesn't have taste buds, so the treat
of a flavoured condom is wasted.

10 Orgasm

The human orgasm is still a modern marvel, even though this phenomenon of ecstatic sexual pleasure has now been examined and analysed in numerous experiments and studies.

An orgasm is best described as an intense pleasurable feeling at the climax of sexual activity. An orgasm is accompanied by involuntary muscle contractions and leads to the release of sexual tensions. In men it is normally accompanied by an ejaculation of semen. To be sexually satisfied, you need to orgasm at least two or three times per week. If masturbation is your only means of sexual relief, you need to orgasm even more often, as the relief it brings is not as intense and won't last as long.

When Irish men have sexual intercourse 83% of them have an orgasm most of the time, but only 65% of Irish women achieve one. That leaves almost two out of every ten men and one out of every three women without the pleasure of climaxing regularly. In men, alcohol plays a huge role in failing to orgasm, as well as medical conditions like diabetes, or mental stress that can be caused by problems at work. A new relationship or a background of bad experiences, are also factors. Women often don't orgasm because they receive much less direct stimulation during intercourse and need a helping hand to climax.

Achieving an Orgasm

Our multi-choice survey revealed that according to couples in Ireland the best ways to achieve an orgasm are as follows:

Women	Total
Intercourse	25%
Intercourse with simultaneous manual stimulation	22%
Masturbation	20%
Cunnilingus	17%
Mutual manual stimulation	16%

Men	Total
Intercourse	41%
Fellatio	20%
Masturbation	17%
Intercourse with simultaneous manual stimulation	12%
Mutual manual stimulation	9%

WOMEN

It's physically more difficult for women to achieve an orgasm during intercourse, as their stimulation is less direct than a man's stimulation of his penis. Women have to try much harder to find sexual satisfaction. The best technique to make a woman come is to manually stimulate her clitoris during intercourse. That's easy to do when she sits on top of you or when you lie behind her. The only problem is that the man has to hold back for at least 12 minutes, as his level of arousal is usually well ahead of his partner's, especially if he didn't do something to cool himself down during foreplay.

'At first I was embarrassed to ask my fiancé to touch me there when we make love, but our lovemaking is so much better now. I want to sleep with him more often, and come almost every time. It gives him more pleasure as well, he often says that there's no better sensation than feeling me shivering and shaking in his arms when I come. Although, he has to hold still a couple of times when we do this, otherwise he would still come well before me,' Agnes (26) from Co. Dublin.

Only one out of every four Irish women (25%) can achieve an orgasm with intercourse alone.

'I have never had a problem coming,' tells Mary (18), from Co. Kerry 'it just happened like clockwork from the very first time. But from talking to my friends, I'm aware that I'm extremely lucky in this regard; they all envy me.'

One out of every six women (17%) comes best when her partner performs cunnilingus.

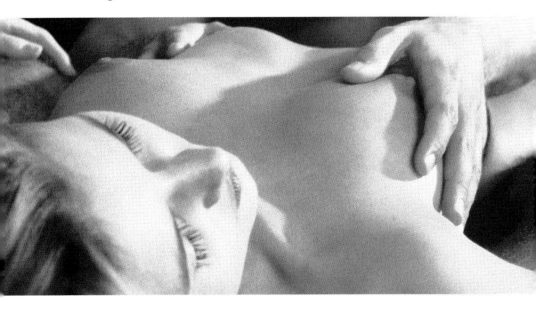

'He starts teasing the tip of my clitoris tenderly with his tongue, then starts circling movements around my pleasure spot, increasing his pressure expertly, at last gently sucking. We have been practising this love game for the last four years, reading countless sex books and trying out everything else. It's the only guaranteed way to make me come,' explains Elaine (37) from Co. Laois. 'And the best thing is that I am under no pressure, but can take all the time I need, as he patiently waits for his turn to be spoiled later.'

The results show that one out of three Irish women (36%) climax best when they either masturbate or have their partner stimulate them manually. Add to those figures the 22% of women who need manual stimulation during intercourse, and you end up with well over half of all Irish women (58%) needing some sort of manual stimulation to achieve an orgasm.

MEN

Irish men find it easiest to come when they have normal intercourse (41%), with fellatio being the second favourite (20%). The figures for fellatio would be dramatically higher, if women didn't give up too soon when they are spoiling their lovers orally. For a man to climax by fellatio takes much longer than climaxing during intercourse.

'It is a completely different type of arousal,' explains Derek (29) from Co. Dublin. 'When you have intercourse, you are in charge of the situation. You know how to move and get excited. It is completely different with fellatio. Sure, you're excited as hell when she puts her lips around you, but then she doesn't find the right rhythm, keeps scraping your penis shaft with her teeth, or doesn't apply enough pressure. In the end, it's the best orgasm ever, if she didn't give up on you before you managed to come.'

One out of every six Irish guys (17%) comes best when he masturbates, and for an additional nine per cent masturbation by their partner is the best method of climaxing. Added up, that amounts to one out of four guys (26%) who have the best chances of getting an orgasm when they are manually stimulated. Another 12 per cent prefer intercourse with simultaneous manual stimulation – that leaves us with a total of 38 per cent who need to be touched. So hands on, ladies.

'When I get a chance to sleep with my girlfriend, it is normally under conditions that are far from ideal,' explains Peter (19) from Co. Mayo. 'It could be in the car or on the couch on a night when my parents are out. I just can't relax enough to come under those conditions, with both of us being naked, and the risk that somebody might walk in on us any moment. And on top of that I'm still inexperienced and a bit clumsy, not knowing what exactly to do during intercourse. So the best way for me to come is still by masturbation. Most of the time I do it on my own, but sometimes my girlfriend gives me a hand, and that makes it much more exciting.'

What If He Fails To Come?

If your man fails to climax when you have sex, stimulate his testicles and anus with your hands, massage his buttocks, kiss his neck, try a bit of dirty talk. If it doesn't work, don't make him try harder, but encourage him to relax. He can keep on stimulating you with his hands and mouth while he takes a break. Pushing him too hard increases the risk of him loosing his erection, and that definitely doesn't help. With a wilting erection, so goes his self-confidence, and then you may as well call it a night.

The best thing for a guy to do in that situation is to concentrate on satisfying his partner. Move in place with your hands and lips and try to give her an orgasm that way. If you hit the right spots and manage to make her come, that takes a lot of pressure off you, and more likely than not you will be able to climax yourself afterwards.

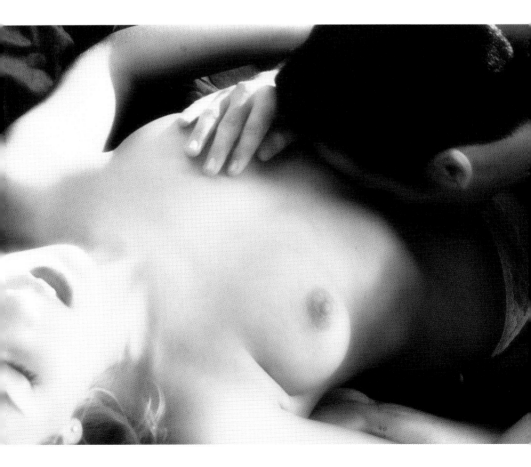

Faking It

Only four out of ten Irish women (40%) and eight out of ten Irish men (80%) never fake an orgasm. Men are naturally much better off when it comes to achieving a real orgasm. However one out of 20 Irish guys has severe problems climaxing and, much to their distress, it shows. It is pretty tough for a guy, especially for a young guy, to pretend that he has come. It's not only the unmistakable lack of semen. A woman can feel the ejaculation pulsing through his penis. For many women, that's the most intimate and enjoyable part of sleeping together. Some women hold still when the moment has finally come and climax when their partner's semen floats into them.

A woman can fake an orgasm quite easily. All she has to do is go to the trouble of first analysing and then faking all the obvious signs, especially the vaginal contractions, that accompany a real orgasm.

Seven per cent of women and five per cent of men fake an orgasm always or most of the time during intercourse. The main reasons are to please your partner, not to disappoint him or her, feeling embarrassed, or simply the wish to get the act over with. It is okay to fake an orgasm occasionally, but don't let it become a habit.

Multiple Orgasms

While many women struggle to climax at least once, some manage to achieve multiple orgasms – that means two or more orgasms in rapid succession. Multiple orgasms very rarely occur in men, it's mainly women who enjoy them. To make a woman come more often than once an intensive foreplay is essential. Tease her until she's almost ready to come, but pull back before it happens, then start again. Slip inside her when she's about to climax. Keep moving when she has her orgasm, and simultaneously caress her clitoris. With a bit of luck you might succeed in spoiling her with a multiple orgasm.

FAKING

Acting like you have had an orgasm when you have not.

MULTIPLE ORGASMS

Achieving two or more orgasms in rapid succession during one sex session.

ORGASM

An intense pleasurable feeling at the climax of sexual activity. It's accompanied by involuntary muscle contractions and leads to the release of sexual tensions. In men, an orgasm is normally accompanied by the ejaculation of semen.

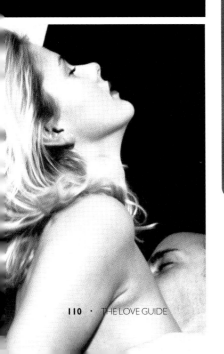

Ireland's Orgasm Survey:

How often do you orgasm during intercourse?

	WOMEN	MEN
Always	16%	58%
Most of the time	49%	25%
50/50	17%	12%
Rarely	11%	4%
Never	7%	1%

How often do you fake an orgasm during intercourse?

	WOMEN	MEN
Always	2%	1%
Most of the time	5%	4%
Sometimes	12%	5%
Rarely	41%	10%
Never	40%	80%

How do you express your orgasm?

	WOMEN	MEN
Moan	69%	68%
Cry out	17%	16%
Bite and scratch	23%	12%
Cry	6%	2%
Stay still	15%	22%
Almost pass out	10%	8%

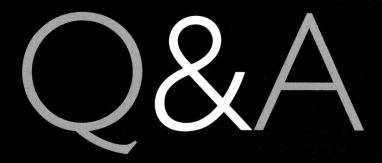

She never has an orgasm when we sleep together - how can I make her come?

Spend a lot of time on foreplay before you make love. Start kissing and teasing her, then massage her clitoris with light circling movements. Be very gentle at first, then gradually apply a bit more pressure and let your hand move faster. Observe her reaction to make sure she enjoys what you're doing. When she's almost ready to come, start making love. Keep caressing her clitoris while you are inside her. It is not easy to find the right touch, so ask her how she would like to be caressed if you don't manage to find out on your own.

What is the best position for a woman to achieve an orgasm?

It is not so much the position that counts, but the right technique. It is easier for a woman to achieve an orgasm when her partner caresses her clitoris before and during intercourse. This works best when she either sits on top or he takes her from behind.

Is it okay to fake an orgasm?

It is okay to fake an orgasm now and then to please your partner, but you should never let it become a habit. There is no point in constantly deceiving your man by letting him believe your sex life is satisfying. Instead of faking an orgasm, give your partner the chance to make you truly happy in bed. Let him know how you like being caressed and kissed. He depends on your feedback to learn how to satisfy you.

I never reach an orgasm when I sleep with my husband, so I secretly masturbate after he has fallen asleep.

Don't feel bad for masturbating after your husband has left you unsatisfied. But to make your sex life more satisfying, you need to let your husband know that you don't come when you sleep with him. Tell or show him how he can stimulate you during intercourse to help you to reach an orgasm.

I have been faking an orgasm since I got married, but I can't do it anymore. The problem is how can I tell my husband that I have never had an orgasm when he made love to me?

I don't think it is a good idea to let your husband know that you have been faking your orgasm all the time. He would not only be disappointed, but probably be angry with you as well. Instead, just stop faking. Make your husband caress your clitoris when you make love, that will help you to come for real. If you have any other ideas about what he could do for you, don't hesitate to let him know.

What is the difference between a clitoral and a vaginal orgasm?

The difference between a clitoral and a vaginal orgasm is not about where you feel your climax; it is about where you are being stimulated. A vaginal orgasm is caused by penetration alone, while a clitoral orgasm occurs due to direct stimulation of the clitoris. But however you achieve your orgasm, the clitoris plays a central role.

My girlfriend makes a lot of fuss when we have sex. She moans plenty, squeaks and sometimes even screams, when she comes. The problem is I very much doubt that she ever really had an orgasm when we made love. She behaves so unnaturally that I'm afraid she's only faking it. How can I tell the difference?

A female orgasm mainly shows in three ways: hard breathing, increased heartbeat and vaginal contractions. While it's easy to fake the first two signs, it's more difficult with the third. If your girlfriend has an orgasm, you should feel her vagina contracting about ten times. But even that isn't a sure sign. If a woman is good at faking, it's almost impossible to tell the difference. The best way to tell for sure whether your girl normally fakes her orgasm or not, is to try especially hard to make her come 'for real'. Caress her clitoris with your hand while you make love to her, as most women find it much easier to come that way.

My boyfriend obviously has had previous girlfriends who went wild when they had their orgasm, shouting and screaming. I'm completely different. When I come, I'm quiet and calm, and hold him tight, not moving at all. He accuses me of only faking an orgasm and lying to him about it.

There are many more ways to enjoy an orgasm than shouting and screaming. Moans and gasps are more common but some women like the quiet way, holding their partner tight and enjoying the close and intense intimacy of the moment. If anything, shouting and screaming sounds like faking, as that's the way orgasms are mainly presented in porn films.

My girlfriend is very noisy in bed, she moans a lot when we make love, getting louder and louder, until she starts crying out shortly before she comes. Her climax is finally accompanied by a piercing scream. Our next door neighbours are an elderly couple who have repeatedly woken up when we made love. A couple of times they've banged on the bedroom wall we share, shouting for us to stop the noise. My friend says not to worry, she's entitled to make as much noise in bed as she wants to. Although I don't want to spoil her fun, I can see our neighbours' point as well. Is there any way to satisfy both?

The best thing to do is to come to a compromise. Let your friend have her way when it's not too late at night. When you feel like making love in the middle of the night, ask her to be a bit more discreet, or try to smother her cries with kisses. And why not move to another room farther away from your neighbours' bedroom once in a while? Your neighbours will appreciate it, and on top it's a nice change for yourselves.

The only problem I have with my girlfriend is that she always bites my neck when she comes. We both love nibbling and biting during intercourse, but her orgasm bite is so strong that she leaves marks on my neck all the time. You can imagine the amount of slagging I get over it. I would hate to ask her to stop biting me, although it sometimes hurts too much for my taste. What can I do about this?

Ask your girlfriend to sink her teeth into another part of your body when she comes. She could bite your shoulder. It probably won't hurt less, but at least then her bite marks would be less visible to others. Another solution would be to make love in positions that don't allow her to bite you, like making love from behind.

I enjoy making love, but I have never come. I have never come in my life, so I don't really know what is supposed to happen. My body starts to shake but then I still don't come. My boyfriend says I need to just relax, but I am relaxed. I just wish I could come for him as it makes him feel bad that he can't make me climax. Could you describe what is meant to happen? I know when men come they ejaculate sperm. Does anything come out of us as well?

From the way you describe your feelings, I'd say you are almost there. It is impossible to give an exact description of the female orgasm, but there are some typical physical indicators. The main signs of sexual excitement are an increased lubrication of the vagina, an increased heartbeat and much quicker breathing. The climax finally shows in involuntary contractions of the vaginal muscle, accompanied by pleasant shudders. Unlike men, women don't ejaculate, although some expel a small amount of fluid when their vaginal muscle contracts. But all in all, a woman's orgasm is less obvious than a man's.

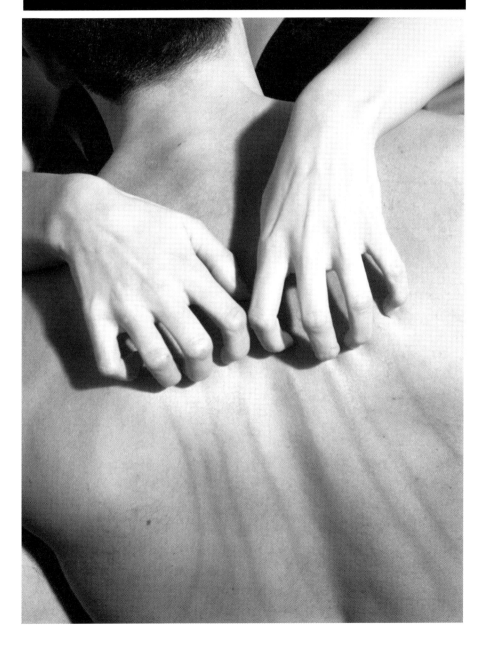

Love Talk

Thankfully the times are over when love and sex were topics you didn't talk about – not even with your partner.

There are still many old inhibitions that keep us in their grip, but their impact keeps getting weaker. There are many reasons to talk about love and sex. For a happy love life it's vital that you express your feelings, and that you talk about your wishes and fantasies. There are many ways to do this – let's have a closer look.

Declarations of Love

'I love you' is by far the most appreciated declaration of love all over the world. These three simple words, that mean so much, are the most basic, and at the same time the most intimate, way to declare your love. Verbal declarations of love are, of course, only one of many ways to show your feelings. You can prove your love in many other ways, but it's still important to say it out loud from time to time.

If you are too shy to tell your partner that you love them face-to-face, leave a voice message, or if you are not up to that either, send a text. In time, you'll have to improve your technique, but in the beginning the most important thing is that he or she gets the message. After that it gets tricky. For a woman you can't say 'I love you' too often. But with men you have to be careful not to overdo it, otherwise they might feel trapped by the threat of too much commitment and responsibility.

'My girlfriend literally smothered me with her love,' explains Alan (41) from Co. Sligo. 'She rang me several times a day to say I love you, and when she couldn't reach me she left a voice message or sent a text. If she had done it just a couple of times per week that would have been great, but I simply couldn't stand it several times per day. I switched my phone off, but then I had to deal with all her voice and text messages later on. It was just too much.'

So declare your love, but don't overdo it!

Don't think that there is no need to say 'I love you' anymore just because your partner knows that you love him or her anyway. Knowing isn't the point. To be happy and content, and to feel safe in a relationship, people need constant reassurance.

The exact choice of words is up to you – tell your guy you're mad about him; assure your girlfriend that she is the woman of your dreams. Find other, playful and colourful ways to articulate your love. Read a love poem. Or why not sing a love song? Even if you are a far cry from ever hitting the charts, it's going to be appreciated.

'My boyfriend surprised me with a love poem on the night we first made love. We were cuddling and teasing, and when I thought it was going to happen, he stopped and said that he had to tell me something first. Then he got this crumpled up piece of paper out of his back pocket, unfolded it and started to read it out. It was a love poem he'd written himself. That was the sweetest way a guy has ever expressed his love for me.' Sinead (19) from Co. Kilkenny.

Wishes and Fantasies

It is important to always have an open mind about your partner's wishes, especially sexual ones. You also need to express your own wishes and fantasies. Many couples miss out on the chance to have more fun together because they are shy or embarrassed. So share your sexual fantasies with your partner. There is a good chance that there is some wish or fantasy that both of you are dreaming about, but are too shy to talk about. Don't sit down for a serious chat; mention your fantasies in a playful way to check out how your partner feels about them.

However you approach it, the main point is to share. Once you have tried it out, you will see how arousing it can be to talk about all the things you fancy.

'It took me three years to make my wife talk about what she likes in bed, and what I might do better. Since she shared her fantasies and wishes with me, our sex life is much better than before. I had no idea that she fancied trying out sex toys, or wanted to make love on the beach. There are so many pleasures we would have missed out on if she hadn't opened up. But it is not only our sex life that has improved, our relationship has become even deeper and more intimate since we started talking about it.' Ian (36) from Co. Cavan.

Compliments

You can never give too many compliments. Tell your partner in detail and at length what you love about them. Compliment their best bodily assets, especially when you are making love. Tell them how great they look, how pleasant they smell, how good it feels to touch them. Make encouraging comments when you are in bed together to spur your partner on. It can be a simple 'you're great' or 'oh, I love this', if you can't think of anything more elaborate at that moment.

'My husband isn't great with words when it comes to showing his feelings,' says Joanna (28) from Co. Dublin. 'He is too shy to even moan when we make love. But when I treat him to something special, like oral sex, he grunts something like "oh yeah babe". It sounds stupid now that I'm telling it, but in bed it's completely different. I see it as a compliment – as his appreciation of my efforts.'

Take an interest in your partner's looks. Keep your eyes peeled to watch out for new items of clothing, a new haircut, even a small change in make-up style. Although you should only compliment what you like, it's important to let your partner know that you notice even the slightest change in their appearance.

Erotic Whispers

Erotic whispers are a great turn on, not only in bed. It can be something harmless like, 'You look so sexy, I'd love to take you home straightaway', when you are just entering a pub or arriving at a party, or you can try something juicy and more explicit that makes your partner blush.

'My girlfriend is great at making me horny with her sexual whispers,' tells George (31) from Co. Waterford. 'She loves to do it in public, when we are out for a drink, or sometimes even when we are in town shopping. She just leans over towards me and whispers into my ear that she would love to see me naked or that she'd love to drag me into the nearest alleyway. The other day we were in the pub, and she asked me to get an erection for her on the spot to show that I still fancy her. It only took me a few seconds... '

Arousing your partner in public has the special kick that goes with doing something outrageous in front of other people. If you imagine that anybody could overhear your whispers it makes them more exciting. To know that the erotic promises can't be fulfilled until you're safely home is also an exquisite torture.

'He whispered all these erotic things into my ear at a party,' admits Rachel (32) from Co. Dublin. 'Like how he loves the way my breasts brush against his body. Then he started to discreetly nibble on my ear, while talking about where else on my body he'd love to put his lips. It was such a turn on that we had to stop the car on our way home. We made love right there in the car, something we hadn't done since we first started dating years ago.'

You shouldn't be too shy to share your feelings – especially in bed.

I love to feel the light tingle of my husband's lips against my ear when he is whispering what he is going to do with his hands and lips in a few moments.' Irene (26) from Co. Longford.

Whisper into her ear how great it feels to be deep inside her; tell him how extraordinarily big he feels when you make love in the morning. Check out your partner's reaction to see how far you can go as there are a good few of us who not only love harmless erotic whispers, but much more explicit erotic talk as well.

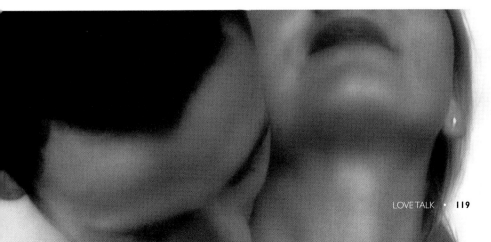

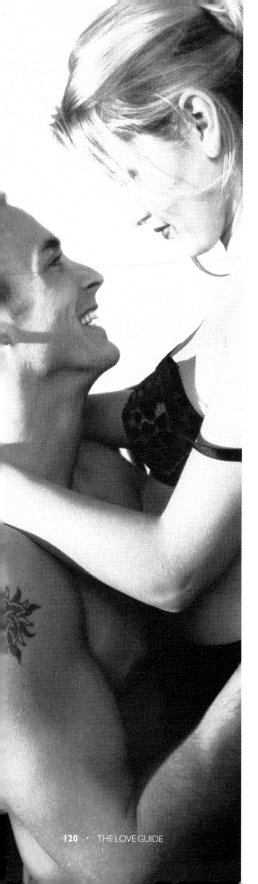

Talking Dirty

How do you feel about talking dirty? Do you love to whisper naughty words into your partner's ear? Do you wish your partner would talk about their lust and love more openly, using explicit vocabulary to express their feelings and wishes?

Talking dirty used to be only appreciated by men, but that is changing rapidly. More and more women like to talk dirty, and to hear naughty stuff from their men as well. Just to make sure: talking dirty doesn't mean tender whispers of love, but using sexy, explicit, naughty language.

If you aren't sure what your partner thinks about talking dirty, but long to give it a try, take it easy at first. Start by using tame language. Tell your girl how you spent all day longing to be inside her. Let your guy know how you wanted to feel him inside you all day. If that doesn't scare her or him off, get more explicit and describe, in detail, what you have in mind. If that goes down smoothly as well, feel free to whisper and groan words and phrases you were taught to never ever let pass your lips.

'When my wife and I first started to talk dirty it wasn't much more than shy whispers that passed our lips. But over the years we have progressed to getting very explicit. My wife's favourite is to talk dirty to me when we are out of the house. She turns me on with descriptions of how she is going to take me into her mouth, letting me know every detail, knowing how much I love it, and how much I suffer from not getting it right now. But later on when we are in bed together, she never lets me down, she always fulfils her promises.' Bert (43) from Co. Offaly.

When you play the bad girl/bad boy game, or use really dirty language that would be insulting under normal circumstances, make sure that your partner knows that you are only play-acting, living out a fantasy, while in real life you respect them. Draw the line at saying anything that makes your partner feel seriously offended.

The most appreciated dirty talk is words of praise and encouragement. Verbal proof of sexual desirability tops the list. For guys, this mainly means appreciation of their potency. If you let men know how great they are it actually helps them to be more potent. This especially works for inexperienced men, but it also helps guys who are making love to a new partner for the first time, or who are worried about not being good enough, or of doing something wrong, or even terrified that they might lose their erection for some reason. Some dirty talk can boost their self-esteem and therefore their potency as well. Again, don't start with language that would make a sailor blush. Tame language is best at the beginning – you can always build on that if it turns your partner on.

'My boyfriend was extremely nervous and embarrassed about being inexperienced the first time we made love. When I felt him struggle to keep his erection, I encouraged him with some dirty talk. He immediately forgot about his worries, and we had a wonderful night.' Davina (27) from Co. Carlow.

If your partner loves talking dirty, give him or her explicit descriptions of your sexual wishes and intentions. Describe in detail how you are going to take them, how you're going to move your head down to let your tongue play with their intimate parts. Find other expressions for dull sounding words like penis and vagina. It's no big turn on to tell your girl: 'I'm going to put my penis into your vagina'. Be experimental and play with words. Use expressions that you have read somewhere, be inventive and use your imagination to think of hot new words.

If you are normally too shy to express your sexual wishes in bed, talking dirty might be the solution for you. When you are playing and acting, it's much easier to say sexy and naughty things that under normal circumstances would never pass your lips.

Sex Instructions

One out of four Irish men likes being told what to do in bed. So ladies don't be shy, try it out. Tell him exactly how you want him to spoil you. Try the game of being dominant; let him, playfully, be your sex slave and demand that he listen to your instructions. Change roles to be fair and let your partner have a go at his secret fantasies. Let him describe them first in detail.

'My man absolutely loves it when I take over and tell him what to do,' tells Sarah (37) from Co. Mayo. 'We often start this game long before we go to bed. He loves to hear me talking dirty. I start winding him up while we have dinner, then he has to do the dishes while I give him instructions for our sex session later on.'

Guys have to be a bit more careful when they play such games with their lovers. One out of five women loves to get instructions, but they better be delivered in a respectful way if you don't want to put her off.

What Irish Women Want to Hear:

Declarations of Love	49%
Encouraging Compliments	48%
Erotic Whispers	46%
Lustful Moans	39%
Dirty Talk	28%
Sex Instructions	21%
Sexual Fantasies	8%
Wild Cries of Lust	7%

What Irish Men Want to Hear:

Lustful Moans	38%
Dirty Talk	37%
Erotic Whispers	35%
Wild Cries of Lust	34%
Encouraging Compliments	33%
Sexual Fantasies	29%
Sex Instructions	27%
Declarations of Love	18%

TIPS

Put Your Feelings into Words
Tell your partner how much you love him or her. Don't assume it's not necessary just because they know how you feel.

Moan and Groan
In bed, reward your partner's efforts with verbal declarations of lust and satisfaction as well as lustful moans and groans.

Declare Your Love, But Don't Overdo It

SEX DICTIONARY

EROTIC
Regarding sexual love and desire. From the Greek word eros, meaning sexual love.

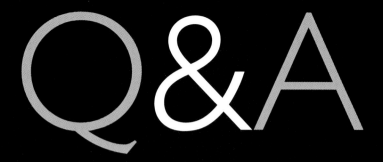

Q&A

My husband and I love to talk dirty on the phone. We ring each other at work, and enjoy having our sex chat. Is it normal to do this?

A bit of phone sex is a great way to brighten up your day. It is absolutely normal, and I can't see any reason why you shouldn't enjoy it.

My wife of 20 years keeps asking me whether I still love her. Of course I do, and she knows that. So why does she keep asking?

Even if you know that your partner loves you, or at least are pretty sure that he does, it is reassuring and comforting to hear him say it. So don't wait for your wife to ask for confirmation, just tell her now and then on your own initiative.

I love to talk dirty in bed, but my boyfriend says he hates women being vulgar, and wants me to stop. Our love life could be much nicer if he would play along instead of shutting me up. How can I make him understand that?

Try a compromise. He can't expect you to shut up in bed, but you could at least refrain from using obscene language, as vulgarity obviously turns him off. Talk sexy instead of dirty, and your boyfriend might even learn to enjoy it.

My boyfriend talks dirty when we make love. I told him that I feel insulted by the vulgarities he utters, but he says that I'm inhibited, and should talk dirty in bed myself, but I could never bring myself to say such vulgar things.

Your boyfriend doesn't mean to hurt you when he talks dirty in bed – he uses vulgarities merely to increase his lust – not to insult you. If you feel offended ask him to be less explicit. Of course you don't have to talk dirty yourself if you don't want to. Your boyfriend should be content with a compromise: let him talk dirty if it turns him on so much, but under the condition that he doesn't expect you to do the same.

I can only see my boyfriend the odd weekend, as we live far apart. So at least once a week we talk dirty on the phone while we touch ourselves – it's the only way for us to be intimate. Although I enjoy it, I still feel a bit uneasy doing this. Is it normal to have sex over the phone? Or should we stop?

There is no reason why you should stop it, whether it's normal or not. You don't see much of each other, so phone sex is the only way you can enjoy your love life together during the week. That is far better than being sexually frustrated altogether.

I would love to talk dirty to my husband, to whisper erotic things into his ear, and to tell him what I'd love him to do with me. But how would my husband react? We are both very shy in bed, and never say a word.

Give it a try, there is a good chance that your husband will love it, especially when you praise or encourage him. But for starters, better be careful. Begin with sexy whispers. Depending on how your husband reacts, you can become bolder in time.

12 One-Night Stand

One-night stands are spontaneous sexual adventures without any further commitment than two people enjoying a night of passion together. The point is to be wild, and to share a good dose of passionate sex together without having to bother about any consequences. Most couples say goodbye the morning after, and that's it.

Sex is the magic word. The pure desire for sex is the main motivation that makes people look for a one-night fling. These men and women don't want to have to wait until they have found the right partner, and then have to patiently wait some more until the relationship has come to the stage where sex starts being an option – they want to fulfil the urge right now. A one-night stand sounds like the perfect solution. Curiosity is part of the game as well: what does it feel like to be intimate with a stranger, without being in love?

More than every second Irish man (57%) and four out of ten Irish women (40%) have had one-night stands. Most of them have had far more than one. Their memories of these flings are about exceptionally good sex and great fun. The majority have thoroughly enjoyed their one-night of 'no strings attached' passion.

'I have always had fantastic sex when I went for a one-night stand,'
explains Nora (24) from Co. Leitrim. 'I always choose my partner
carefully, making sure that he's sober enough and doesn't take any drugs.
When we're finally in bed together, I forget about all the inhibitions and
restraints I feel with a steady partner. I just do whatever I feel like,
without the slightest embarrassment.'

Let's have a closer look at what's so special about one-night stands – what makes them rate higher on the lust scale than the average night with your partner?

The Pros

Excitement of the 'First Time'
Every one-night stand is a 'first time', with all the new excitement of seeing the person naked, of exploring their body, and of feeling them intimately – something never experienced before.

You all know the feeling of being shy around a new lover, and remember the excitement of the very first touches, and the first deep kiss. Then the tingle of the first caresses, the first time he brushes his hand against her breast, or the first time he feels her hand on his penis. Then the longing for more and the long wait until you finally get to make love. In a relationship it can take months before you first sleep together but the unspoken rule of a one-night stand is to have sex almost straight away. Everything from flirting to having sex happens at high speed. You might start off feeling a little bit shy, but then you'll usually get carried away by your lust and end up jumping into bed.

2 Lack of Restraints

The mutual agreement in a one-night stand is to share a night of sex and fun. Restraints — if you have any — are left behind. One-night stands are the ideal playground for your hidden fantasies and wishes. It is often so much easier to try out new tricks, ideas and techniques with a complete stranger. You can live out your dreams with a partner who is just as eager as you are to try anything new.

If you make a fool of yourself or have second thoughts the next day, that's no big deal, as you'll probably never see them again.

'Whenever I feel kinky I go out to catch a guy for a one-night stand,' admits Barbara (28) from Co. Dublin. 'I dress up sexily, get some fun condoms, and sometimes even pocket a small sex toy, like my vibrator lipstick. Then I live out my fantasies without having to worry about the next day. Most of the time I don't stay until the morning anyway, but sneak out before he wakes up.'

3 Feeling of Being Naughty

It can be such a turn on to be naughty. The knowledge of doing something forbidden makes whatever you're up to just that little bit more exciting. And, although one-night stands are regarded as almost normal sexual behaviour nowadays, they still have a touch of being bad.

'I like being bad now and then,' admits Rhonda (19) from Co. Dublin. 'Life is boring if you stick strictly to the rules all the times. If I listened to my parents, I would still be a virgin waiting to be brought in front of the altar before I had sex. I listen to them most of the time, but not when it comes to sex. I prefer to go steady with a boy, but whenever I'm single, I go for one-night stands to get what I need.'

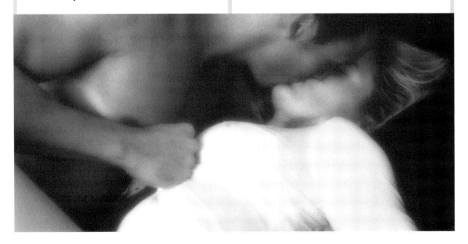

The Cons

Although one-night stands are regarded as great fun most of the time, they can have a dark side as well. I'd say it's best to think about the cons for a second before you jump into an adventure unprepared.

In the worst-case scenario, one-night stands can turn nasty. So it's important that you feel comfortable and secure enough with your lover. It is often safer for a woman to bring a man back to her house or flat, especially if she shares her pad with flatmates. If possible, always let a person you trust know where you are and what you are up to. Always remember to use condoms – to be extra careful always carry your own pack.

Here are some common complications that you should be aware of:

▌ Falling in Love *Falling in love is problem number one. Experiencing sudden strong feelings of love the next day is a real nuisance, especially if only one person feels them. After all, the unspoken deal was to spend a passionate night together – without commitment and complications.*

You don't want to wake up, realising that you have fallen in love, only to be handled like any other one-night stand by your newly beloved. And if you are the one who plays it cool and sticks to the rules, you don't want your one-night stand partner to cling to you once the night is over.

If you would love to see your fling again, there is nothing wrong with giving him or her your phone number. But it's not a good idea to ask for theirs. Leaving your number is an unmistakable sign that you would like to see him or her again. So leave it up to them whether they want to make the call.

'I can't stand it when a woman asks for my number,' complains Niall (29) from Co. Kerry. 'I have had some really bad experiences in that regard, like getting calls and messages all the time. If a woman wants to see me again, she can leave her number, and I might ring her back, although most of the time I wouldn't. Meeting for a second time is almost like starting a relationship, and I don't want any commitment at the moment.'

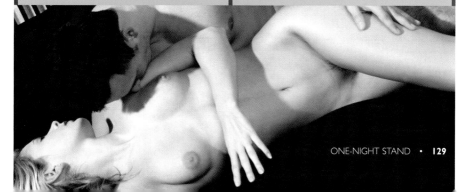

There are some scenarios that can leave you with a bad aftertaste. The most common is to be hit by a bad conscience the morning after. Especially if you have been on the fling while your loving and caring partner has been waiting for you at home.

Waking up with a hangover beside someone you would never go near in your right state of mind is another nightmare you could do without.

And finally, you might get hit by a panic attack when you realise that you have had unprotected sex with a complete stranger. To avoid this drama, you should make it your first priority to always use condoms when you have a one-night stand. Play it safe and get them yourself. Don't expect your fling to look after protection.

Too Impersonal
Some people realise that one-night stands are too impersonal after all. They feel hurt being treated like sex objects, and miss the love and care they feel with a steady partner. Their solution – never do it again. Although most give it another chance once the bad feelings have abated.

'My worst experience was with a guy who asked me to get up and leave his place as soon as he had climaxed. I have had many flings, but had never seen anything like this before. I felt so humiliated, I was in tears when I slammed the door behind me,' Monica (33) from Co. Meath.

TIPS

Always use condoms when you have a one-night stand.

Choose a partner when you are sober.

Don't ask them: 'Do you love me?'

Don't cling to your fling afterwards. Clinging is the worst sin of a one-night stand.

If you wish to see your fling again, give him or her your number, but don't ask for theirs.

Ireland's One-Night Stand Survey Results:

WHAT DID YOU LIKE?

	WOMEN	MEN
The excitement of the 'first time'	41%	26%
The lack of restraint	24%	32%
The feeling of being naughty	23%	25%

WHAT DID YOU DISLIKE?

	WOMEN	MEN
I fell in love	28%	10%
The aftermath	23%	14%
It was too impersonal	22%	18%
Partner clinged to me, wouldn't let go	13%	27%

WHAT WAS YOUR SITUATION?

	WOMEN	MEN
He or she just fascinated me	44%	21%
Merely wanted sex	40%	59%
Was drunk	29%	22%
Was tired of relationships	23%	10%

Q&A

I am very casual when it comes to sex. When I fancy a guy I sleep with him, often taking the initiative. The problem is that I only get as far as one-night stands. No man I've ever been with was interested in a serious relationship.

For a serious relationship guys tend to go for women who are harder to get and less fixated on sex. It also doesn't help when you get a reputation for sleeping around. To fulfill your dream of a steady relationship, you should slow down and become a bit more choosy and serious in your love life.

I have had a one-night stand with a man who has a reputation for never sleeping with the same woman twice. I had hoped that it would be different with me, but he refuses to see me again. Not only that, he doesn't even answer my calls. He completely ignores me.

You knew this guy's reputation when you slept with him, so you shouldn't be surprised or disappointed about the way he's treating you. The best way to catch a guy like him is to play hard to get instead of pulling out all the stops. But I find it hard to understand why any woman would want to be with a man who's swapping lovers like underwear. Sure, it's a challenge to coax him into a relationship, but in the end you buy yourself much more trouble and heartache than happiness. So the best you can do is to forget about your one-night stand.

When I had a look at my one-night stand the morning after, I saw that his penis was covered in red blotches. I'm not sure whether he used a condom that night, but I don't think so. I'm worried that he might have infected me with some sexual disease. How long do I have to wait to make sure I didn't catch anything?

You should see a doctor immediately. You can't just wait and sit things out. It can take months, even years, for some infections to show. You have to consult a gynaecologist for a check-up, explaining what happened to give them an idea about what to look for.

I fell in love with my one-night stand, but he refused to give me his phone number. I found it out anyway, but when I sent him a text, the only answer I got was to leave him alone. Why does he have to be so rude?

The best thing you can do is to leave him alone. All you're achieving by trying to contact your fling is to make him annoyed. After all, clinging is the worst sin of a one-night stand. Of course there is nothing wrong with trying to see somebody again, but if this somebody wants to be left alone, it's better to accept that. After all, he had made it clear from the start that he doesn't want to see you again, when he refused to give you his phone number.

Our 18-year-old son often stays away on a Friday or Saturday night. We thought he stayed with a friend, but we have now found out that he's been lying to us. He actually confessed that he goes with girls. Isn't he too young to have one-night stands? We are worried he might get himself into trouble.

Talk to your son. At his age you won't be able to talk him out of sleeping with girls, but you can make sure that he takes all the possible precautions.

13 Sex With The Ex

Sex with an ex-lover is a dangerous game. You have once been in love, and although a lot has happened since then, your feelings could easily overwhelm you again. But in spite of all the risks involved, it is sometimes too tempting to revive an old love story.

If a relationship has been over for a while, it's mainly the good memories that stick in your mind, especially if you feel lonely and badly need some love. Most of all, it's the great times in bed you remember — how perfectly you fit together, and how intimate you were with each others' bodies.

Having sex with your ex can be anything from comforting to passionate, from the best decision of your life to a disastrous mistake. It can set free a roller coaster of emotions.

When it doesn't work out, we excuse ourselves with the fact that we couldn't have known that beforehand. But be honest, most of the time we have a pretty good idea of what we are getting into. The prospect of some good sex with the ex, who knows how to tease and satisfy your sensitive zones to perfection, is just too tempting. And of course there is the silent hope that a night of passion might miraculously bring you back together.

Every second one of us goes back to an ex, and many more have played with the idea. It seems to be almost impossible to get the ex out of our head. It is much more than the wish to return to something and someone familiar. Our ex-lovers have a power over us that is hard to break, even if the relationship was more like a disaster than a dream.

'I let my ex-husband move back in with me, although our marriage had been a nightmare for the past few years,' tells Susan (47) from Co. Dublin. 'He slept around with other women, and finally left me and the kids for one of them. We got a divorce, and shortly afterwards he left his lady friend and came back to the children and me. Everybody said I must be nuts to take him back, but I haven't regretted it yet. We are as happy again as we were at the beginning of our marriage.'

Why Have Sex with the Ex?

The Good Times

Especially at times when we feel lonely, when we have split up with somebody or feel neglected in our new relationship, old memories of the good old times start cropping up. It is so comforting to give in to these memories, and the fact that the ex is only a phone call away can start you thinking. So why not give them a ring to see how they're doing? It's the lonely times like this that make people end up calling their ex-lovers out of the blue. Once you're on the phone, you can't help but reminisce about the old times. So you decide to meet for a drink, for friendship's sake. And then you realise that it still tingles to be near them.

Great in Bed *One of the main reasons why we can't stop thinking about our ex is the fact that the sex was too good to let go. If your ex was great in bed, you inevitably compare all your new lovers with him or her. If you come to the conclusion that no other lover has lived up to them, it is very tempting to revive the old relationship at least on a sexual basis. There is not much harm in that, as long as you keep your emotions in check and don't expect more.*

'Sex was what I missed most after we split up. Now that we live apart and meet strictly for sex, it is even better. There are no more fights, no bad feelings – and a night of very intimate and passionate lovemaking whenever we meet. Nobody knows my body and my needs as well as him,' reveals Annette (34) from Co. Meath.

3 That Tingling Feeling One out of every four of us still feel butterflies when they encounter their ex. The old, initial attraction is still there. The feelings that overwhelm you when you meet your ex again after some time are an enticing mix of old memories of closeness and intimacy, and the thrill of meeting somebody again who is now like a new person.

'When I met my ex again after more than eight years, he had changed so much that I hardly recognised him after he'd spoken the first few words, all those old memories came rushing in. I felt flushed and confused.' Kelly (34) from Co. Dublin.

4 Old Love This is by far the most dangerous reason for clinging to an ex: you still love him or her. This is bad news, for anything less than a real, full relationship wouldn't be good enough for you. You can't be just friends, or have a sexual affair. You would be suffering all the time. One of the worst ideas ever is to coax the ex into bed 'one last time'. It might be comforting for an hour or two, but it is prone to end in misery if you are still in love but your ex doesn't feel the same way.

5 The Ideal Partner Does your ex represent the ideal woman or man for you? Are they exactly the partner you want? If yes, that spells trouble. Idolising an ex doesn't make life easy. By constantly comparing new partners with your ex, you spoil the chance of building up a new relationship. If they are compared with an ex all the time, a new partner doesn't get a real chance to prove that he or she is worth being loved for the person they are. Your new love might be as fantastic as your old one, but in different ways. The problem is that you will never find out as long as you are haunted by the ideal of your ex.

Going for It?

If you still fancy having sex with your ex be honest with yourself about what you really want – is it just sex or do you still hope to renew your relationship? If there is reasonable hope that your ex is still in love with you – give it a try. If not, you should only go for it if you are on the safe side emotionally and sex is all you want. If you wish for more, just be aware that you can't win a person's love back with good sex. Sex, for sure, won't solve any problems that might have occurred between you. If anything, it makes matters worse by adding to your frustration about your broken relationship.

'It took me weeks to realise that my ex had only taken me back because he loved our sex life,' explains Noreen (29) from Co. Westmeath. 'I was still so much in love with him that all I could think about was how good it is to be together again. Then I found out that he was seeing other girls as well. And that was it, I finally left him, being angry not only with my ex but with myself. Our short reunion definitely brought me more grief than pleasure.'

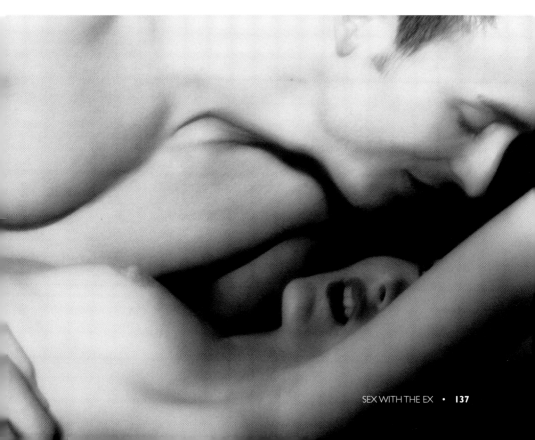

TIPS

Think twice before you make love to your ex again

Go for it if it's just for fun, but be careful if you still love him or her.

Never compare your new love with your ex

Ireland's 'Sex with the Ex' Survey

Did You Ever Have Sex with an Ex?

	WOMEN	MEN
Yes	46%	54%
No	54%	46%

Why Have 'Sex with the Ex'?

	WOMEN	MEN
The good times	47%	54%
Great in Bed	38%	23%
That Tingling Feeling	23%	24%
I still love him/her	8%	12%
He/she is still my ideal	7%	13%

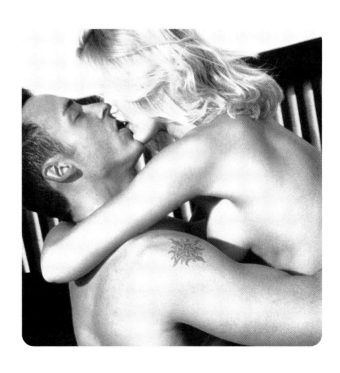

Q&A

On a night out with my old classmates, I flirted with the guy who had been my first love. I hadn't seen him in ten years. We are both married to somebody else now, but I can't stop thinking about him. Should I ring him up?

It is always an emotionally tumultuous event when you meet an ex again, especially after such a long time. All the good memories come flooding back. Don't let that ruin your marriage. Think carefully about what you might be missing in your current partnership, and try to get your marriage back on track instead of chasing an old love.

My boyfriend has started to see his ex again, because I won't sleep with him. I'm only 14, and just don't feel up to it yet. But if I don't sleep with my boyfriend soon, he's going back to his ex.

Don't give in, you are too young to have sex, and your boyfriend has to accept that. If he doesn't, let him go back to his ex. The way he is fooling around with her now to put you under pressure is another good reason why you should end this relationship for good.

I am pregnant by my best friend's ex-boyfriend. We secretly started seeing each other after my best friend dumped him, and he needed a shoulder to cry on. I don't know what to do

Confide in your best friend, I think you should have done that long before now. After all, she has dumped your guy, it's not like you took him away from her. I agree that she won't be happy to see him in your arms, but she'll find out about the two of you anyway, and it's definitely better if she gets the news from you. If she is a true friend, she'll overcome any bad feelings, and will stand by you.

My girlfriend has split up with me, but I can't accept the separation. I still love her very much while she says that she doesn't feel the same for me anymore. I want her anyway, even if she doesn't love me. It hurts, but it's much worse not having her at all.

You have to accept her decision; it's the best for both of you, even if you can't see that at the moment. Being in love with somebody who doesn't feel the same means constantly getting hurt. As long as you stick to this relationship, you deny yourself the chance to fall in love with a girl who loves you back.

My guy never stops comparing me with his ex, who dumped him a while ago. He talks about her all the time, saying she would do this or that now, how she would like the movie we're watching, or how she used to cook her famous Bolognaise. Even in bed he compares me with her all the time. I am really fed up with this. What can I do to make him forget his ex, and enjoy the relationship he has now with me?

Tell your boyfriend about the way you feel. Explain to him that it's okay to mention his ex now and then, but that he needs to stop comparing you with her. You can't be a copy of this other woman, you are your own person, and he should love and accept you the way you are. I'm sure your boyfriend doesn't mean to hurt you, he just hasn't got over the loss of his former girlfriend yet. The fact that he was dumped by her makes it especially hard for him to accept the separation. But he needs to get on and stop brooding about the past.

After splitting up with my last boyfriend, I have finally found the love of my life. He is great all around, except for one thing – he has no skills when it comes to sex. Out of sexual frustration I am seeing my ex again. Now I am torn between the man I love, and my ex who gives me the best sex ever.

Stay with the man you love, and teach him to be a good lover. Tell and show your boyfriend what you like in bed. Not every man has a natural talent to guess a woman's sexual wishes and needs, so you need to let your guy know what you desire.

14 Masturbation

Most people still consider masturbation a taboo subject. Almost everyone does it, but nobody admits it. You can talk about your favourite sex positions or your experience with swinging; discuss your new nipple rings or the merits of bondage but most people find it difficult to talk about the fact that they enjoy masturbating.

We can talk openly about all kinds of sexual matters, but to bring up masturbation is still a guaranteed conversation stopper. All talk will stop, everybody will feel a sudden need to clear their throats, and all eyes will be darting elsewhere hoping to find some excuse to leave. And if somebody has the stomach to ask you out straight, saying something like 'I have always wondered how often you do it', would you give an honest answer? Or would you join the club and try to get off the hook with an entertaining remark that doesn't reveal anything about your own masturbation habits?

So let's start by making a few facts clear: there is nothing wrong with masturbating. It doesn't harm your health, it won't make your penis shrink; it doesn't have any effect on your ability to have children. Masturbation won't give you crooked fingers or a bent spine, you won't run out of sperm and you won't suffer from whatever other afflictions you were told about as a child, to keep you from touching yourself.

Instead of doing you any harm, masturbation has a positive effect on your body. It helps you to relax and to get rid of tension. It is a great method of inducing sleep after a long and stressful day. And it keeps those hormones that keep you happy and content flowing.

More than one out of every four Irish women (28%) and three quarters of all Irish men (75%) masturbate at least a few times per week. Men have a much stronger sex drive than women so it is normal that they masturbate much more often. Most guys even masturbate regularly when they are in a steady relationship, because most women simply don't want sex as often as they do. And again, there is nothing wrong with that. It is the best and easiest way for a couple to stay happy and satisfied together.

Masturbation Techniques

Women

Women normally masturbate by caressing their clitoris. This can be done in many ways. The most promising technique is to apply tender and circling movements around the hot spot itself.

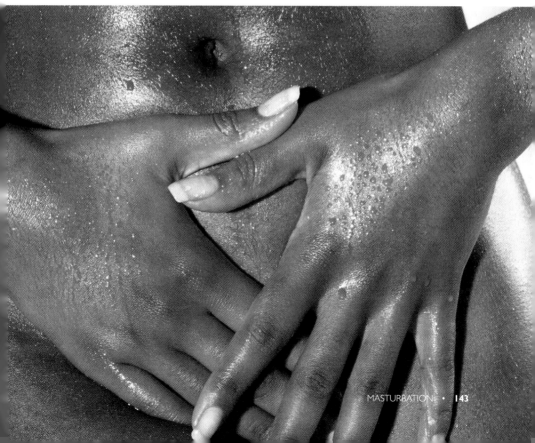

You can also rub off something nice, be it a pillow or your teddy bear, or insert an object into your vagina for stimulation. This can be a vibrator or anything else you might have at hand. If you have nothing else a finger or two should do as well.

Women should never be shy about masturbating. It is a good way of improving your sex life and finding out how to please yourself. After all it's only when you have learned how to pleasure yourself, that you will be able to give your lover directions about what he can do for you.

Men

Most guys masturbate several times a week, or even daily, and that is completely normal. The main technique involved is to simply enclose the penis shaft with your hand and then move your hand up and down to let your foreskin caress the tip of your penis.

If you are circumcised, the technique is a bit trickier. On a circumcised penis, the penis gland is exposed all the time. To make masturbation feel more comfortable on a circumcised member, apply lots of lubricant to make up for the missing foreskin.

Locations

Women and men alike mainly masturbate in the cosy atmosphere of their beds. Two thirds of Irish women (67%) and three quarters of Irish guys (76%) enjoy it in their beds. The bathroom is the second most popular location. One out of three women (33%) and every second man (48%) in Ireland masturbates either in the loo, the shower or the bath. A close third is the sitting room. The car is another popular location, but mainly for young people.

'I often masturbate in my car when I come home from seeing my girlfriend,' admits Kevin (19) from Co. Dublin. 'Sometimes I start while I'm driving, but then I pull over for a minute or two to finish of.'

Not even the workplace is safe – one out of 14 women (7%) and one out of eight men (13%) touch themselves at work. Think about this next time you have a bad day at work – it might help to raise your spirits.

TIPS

There is no harm in masturbating. But if you overdo it, it might leave you sore and will be less satisfying.

Excessive masturbation is not dangerous, but it spoils the fun. If you feel that you don't get much out of masturbation anymore, give yourself a break.

Sex Dictionary

AUTOEROTICISM
Having sex with yourself, like masturbating.

MASTURBATION
Touching one's own genitals to achieve sexual pleasure.

WANK
Slang term for masturbating.

The Irish and Masturbation

HOW OFTEN DO YOU MASTURBATE?

	WOMEN	MEN
At least once per day	10%	25%
A few times per week	18%	50%
Once per week	4%	11%
One to three times per month	22%	8%
Less often	34%	4%
Never	12%	2%

The results of the multi-choice survey revealed:

WHERE DO YOU MASTURBATE?

	WOMEN	MEN
Bed	67%	76%
Bathroom	33%	48%
Sitting room	31%	47%
Car	10%	17%
At work	7%	13%

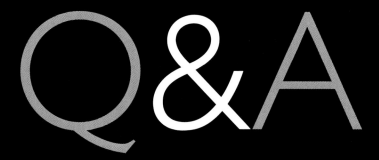

As I don't have a girlfriend yet, I masturbate two to three times per day. Is that dangerous or unhealthy?

There is no harm in masturbating two-three times per day, on the contrary it is very important for your well-being to get sexual relief on a regular basis. Masturbation helps you to relax; it reduces stress, is a very efficient method to induce sleep, releases hormones that ward off depression, and increases the strength of your immune system. In short: masturbating is good for both body and soul.

My husband masturbates on the sly when I don't sleep with him. Why does he do this to me?

What your husband does is only normal. It is his right to play with his own body, whether you sleep with him or not. It has nothing to do with betrayal or unfaithfulness; he is only getting the sexual satisfaction that he needs to be happy and balanced. So let your husband masturbate if he feels like it. If you hate him doing it, you can masturbate him yourself. I'm sure he would appreciate that.

I secretly masturbate after intercourse because my man never makes me come. What if he ever finds out?

There is no need to feel embarrassed about masturbating; you are entitled to look after yourself in bed. But instead of masturbating secretly, you should touch yourself while you make love, or show your partner how you like being caressed down there. You will enjoy your orgasm much more if you can share the experience with your loved one.

Do girls masturbate as well or is it a guys' thing? If girls masturbate – how do they do it?

While guys often talk and brag about their masturbation experiences and even organise competitions to see who performs best, women tend to enjoy auto-erotic pleasures in privacy. Sure, girls masturbate as well, but they do it far less than men. When women masturbate, they normally touch and caress their clitoris until they climax. Some women also like to rub themselves against something nice, like a pillow.

I feel bad for masturbating. Is this normal?

The main reason why people feel bad about masturbating is a bad conscience. Often parents forbid their kids to touch themselves. We grow up hearing that masturbation is sinful and unhealthy. Although as adults we should know better than to believe in these myths, we still half-believe what we have internalized as kids. When you masturbate, you don't do any harm, neither to yourself nor to anybody else. It is your right to find pleasure in your own body, so try to overcome those old inhibitions.

Is it true that masturbating can make your penis shrink? At 15 years of age, I am only about 6½ inches and can't afford to get any smaller. I only masturbate once per week because I'm worried that any more would make my penis shrink. I would cut it out altogether if it would help to maintain its size.

Don't worry, masturbating won't make your penis shrink. So you can do it as often as you like, without the risk of your penis getting smaller. Your penis is a formidable size already, above average for your age, and, as you're only 15, it will probably still gain in size.

Having no girlfriend, I masturbate all the time. This has been going on for years. Can masturbating harm my ability to have children, as I'd love to have children in the future. When I keep touching myself, will my

semen run out so that I can't become a father later in life?

Don't worry, masturbating won't affect your ability to father children in the future. It is an old myth that a man has only a certain amount of 'shots', and then runs out of sperm, but there's no truth in that at all. It's nothing but a myth told to keep boys from masturbating.

Although he has sex with me regularly, my boyfriend (24) still masturbates occasionally. Is that normal, or is something wrong with our relationship? He says he is thinking about me when he touches himself, but I still find it odd. I have to add that we live apart, and only see each other at the weekends. But then we make love two-three times; from what I have heard this is average.

Two-three times per week is the overall average, but couples your age make love more often then that when they have the opportunity. Then, there is a big gap between the sexual needs of men and women. For a guy of 24 it's normal to seek sexual satisfaction daily, so there is nothing wrong or unusual about your boyfriend masturbating when he can't be with you.

15 Pornography

It is no secret that men are by far bigger fans of pornography than women, but women are catching up – slowly but surely. There is nothing wrong with watching porn, as long as you don't get hooked and need it to find sexual satisfaction.

The main difference between the porn preferences of men and women is still the extent of flesh, skin and intimate details exposed. While a woman can easily get carried away by a romantic love story that is only spiced up with a few erotic pictures and scenes, a man normally needs much more explicit stuff to make him aroused and get his lust hormones going.

'I don't care much about the story,' admits Keith (41), 'as long as the women are beautiful and don't hold back with their appeals. All I want to see is sexy women and some sexual action.'

You can find porn in the form of videos, DVDs, books, magazines, and calendars – and of course on the Internet. On the Internet you can find almost anything you can imagine, but you have to be careful about what you choose. The range is impressive but the majority of the offers are not sound and you can get badly ripped off. Some pages are even strictly illegal.

There are two types of pornography. The types are distinguished by how explicit they are in the exposure of intimate details.

Hard-core Pornography

Hard-core pornography is sexually explicit material that graphically shows genitals and sexual acts to stimulate erotic feelings.

Soft-core Pornography

Soft-core pornography is less explicit, sexually arousing depictions or descriptions that leave it up to your imagination and fantasy to fill in the details.

Internet Porn

The availability of pornography on the Internet is like a new playground, that men especially appreciate – it's like all the other new techno gizmos out there.

Being a sexologist, I have to surf the Internet for new inventions and trends all the time. And I can only encourage other women to do the same. Your men are doing it anyway, whether you like it or not. So get ahead of them. Most of what you will find is not worth bothering with, but the odd time you stumble across something that is worth investigating.

If you catch your guy surfing dodgy pages don't worry. There is no harm in getting some inspiration, as long as it doesn't become an obsession. Just make sure you have got the newest anti-virus software installed on your computer before you go surfing for porn, and don't click on any links that suddenly pop up, promising that you have won a great prize and only need to claim it. You need to also be extremely careful when you are being prompted to give your name, address, bank details, or even credit card number to proceed. It could cost you a small fortune.

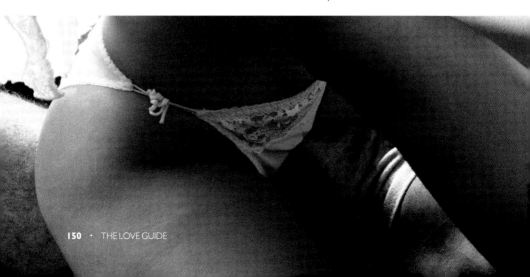

The Porn Factor

Sex videos and DVDs are the most popular ways to view all kind of porn, and the best time to enjoy them is before you have sex. Did you ever watch a porn film with your partner? If not, it is worth a try. Even if an erotic film seems to be a bit foolish, it shouldn't fail to inspire your sexual fantasies.

During Foreplay *Some women enjoy watching soft porn to get them going. The actors should be good-looking, romantic, and masters in the art of seduction. There has to be a story of love and lust behind the action, even if it is something simple or even foolish. Without at least the illusion of some love being involved, women don't get much out of pornography.*

In general men are a bit easier to please. They prefer hard-core porn, not caring much about the content. The main point is that the action is explicit enough, and the close-ups show all the sexy details of lovemaking that you can't observe when you are busy making love yourself.

'I can't help it,' admits Alan (30). 'I just love to watch the details of penetration. The first time I ever saw that was in a porn film. They zoomed in on it, and I got so aroused that I had to masturbate. I still like to watch porn films, but my wife isn't too mad about them. So instead I choose positions that allow me to watch myself penetrating my wife. The best is doggy style; it lets me observe all the details of our lovemaking. And the best thing about it is that my wife can't catch me watching.'

Some men come up with the weirdest sex videos, that often reflect their own secret sexual wishes and fantasies, hoping to maybe awaken the same interest in their girl. Most of the time, this doesn't work. Instead of getting excited, women tend to get the giggles.

Overall men's favourites are porn videos with lesbian scenes and with intimate kisses, especially fellatio. As they watch the actors there is always the hope that their own lover might be tempted to replay a sexy scene if she sees how much it turns her man on. In reality, this seldom works out.

The best approach is to choose a couple of porn films with your partner to satisfy both your tastes. In the beginning it is advisable to choose a well-known brand, to avoid any bad shocks.

2 While You Make Love

One out of every four men and one out of every five women in Ireland loves to watch porn while they make love. It makes lovemaking more interesting and exciting. You not only see erotic postures and scenes on the screen. Next thing – if you play along – they are happening in your own bed.

'That is the best part, to replay the best scenes you have witnessed, while the porn film keeps running in the background, firing you on with it's moans and groans,' describes Barbara (26).

Porn films, books and magazines are a good way to find out more about love, especially the different positions and techniques. Porn videos and DVDs have another advantage as well: they can help men who suffer from potency problems to get and keep an erection. There is no guarantee that it works, but the chances are good, and it is in any case worth a try.

'I find it hard to stay erect when I sleep with my wife,' explains Tony (52). 'She is not very active in bed, and never utters a sound when we sleep together. So I love to have a porn video running in the background. I can have an occasional glimpse at the screen, and can hear all the moaning and dirty talk. My wife didn't like it at first, but she plays along now, as she understands that it helps me to stay potent.'

3 During Masturbation

One of the main functions of porn is to help people, especially men, along when they masturbate. Only one out of seven Irish women (15%), but three out of five Irish men (60%) like to watch porn while they are masturbating. Most men like to start off watching women making love to each other, and then switch to oral love, usually the technique of their dreams: – fellatio.

'I don't have a girl at the moment, but I am very interested in everything that has to do with sex,' explains Duncan (23). 'As masturbation is the only sexual activity I'm getting at the moment, I watch some porn to get my fantasies going. It is so much more fun to imagine that there's this sexy girl from the magazine who has wrapped her hand around my penis. A good trick to make this fantasy more realistic is using my other hand. When I pretend that it's a woman masturbating me, it feels completely different.'

Ireland's Porn Preferences

Which kind of porn do you like?

	WOMEN	MEN
Videos/DVDs	34%	71%
Magazines	21%	35%
Books	13%	14%
Internet	8%	31%

When do you like porn?

	WOMEN	MEN
Having sex with my partner	20%	28%
Before I have sex	29%	59%
While masturbating	15%	60%

Sex Dictionary

HARD-CORE PORN

Sexually explicit material that shows all the intimate details of lovemaking, displaying genitals, penetration, and other sexual acts to stimulate erotic feelings.

SOFT-CORE PORN

Less explicit, sexually arousing depictions or descriptions that need your imagination to fill in the intimate details.

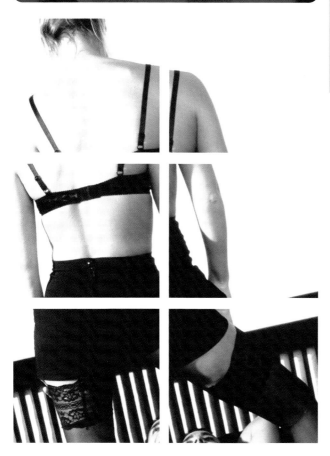

Q&A

My bedroom is decorated with erotic posters, a TV set for watching porn, a variety of sex toys, and a porn collection. The few women I have ever brought home were a bit shocked or even disgusted by this. Now I have met a lady I am really serious about, and I hope to bring her home soon. Will she turn away as the others did when she sees my bedroom?

Your new lady friend will probably find your bedroom decorations and fittings a bit odd to say the least. Your bedroom must look like you are fixated on sex, and that would frighten most women off. Why don't you redecorate a bit? Get some neutral posters, and store away your collection of sex toys and porn.

My boyfriend is reading sex magazines all the time, and doesn't even try to hide it from me. He normally gets aroused, and then expects me to have sex with him. But I can't enjoy making love with him when other women obviously turn him on. He probably even fantasises about the porn girls while I'm in his arms.

It is not so much the girls in those magazines that turn your boyfriend on, but the sexual scenes themselves, so there's no need to be jealous. Did you ever join your boyfriend when he's reading these magazines? It's still mainly a male domain, but statistics show that more and more women are becoming interested, so it might be worth a try. If you are seriously against it, tell your boyfriend that you feel used when he gets turned on by those magazines, and then expects you to fulfil his fantasies.

During all the years of our marriage, I have never observed anything strange about my wife, but now I have caught her watching porn. I was out for the night with some friends, and when I came home earlier than expected, I found my wife in front of the telly, watching an erotic movie and touching herself. I was so shocked and furious that I made a scene, and we haven't talked to each other since. I would forget about the whole thing if she'd apologise, but she says it's me who has to apologise for invading her privacy. It can't go on like this, so can you please tell me what to do?

As your wife didn't do anything wrong don't wait for an apology. In a relationship, both partners need some private space. That goes for yourself as well as for your wife. To end the silence between the two of you, offer a truce. Tell your wife that it's time to deal with this, and that there are two options: to talk about what has happened, and how both of you feel about it, or to just forget about it, and never mention it again. Let your wife then decide what to do.

My husband spends hours every weekend looking up adult pornography on the Internet. When I confronted him, he said he was doing it only out of curiosity. (1) Is this normal behaviour, and (2) is he committing an offence looking up all that sex? I know it's an offence looking up child porn.

To answer your first question, it is normal for a man to show an interest in pornography. In that regard, males are very different from females, which makes it hard for women to understand and accept their men's keen interest in pornographic material. To answer your legal concerns, as far as I know there is no specific law in Ireland related to adult pornography on the Internet, while the general laws about Indecent Publications leave the Internet in a sort of grey zone.

A while ago I saw two girls touching and kissing each other. I found watching them so arousing that I got an erection. This is worrying me, especially as I can't get the picture of those girls out of my head. I'm also curious to know what they get up to in bed with each other. I have to admit that I even bought some porn to find out more about lesbian love. What is wrong with me? I always thought I was normal.

Don't worry, the fascination you feel towards lesbian sexuality is normal. For most men lesbian play is a big turn on, that's the main reason why porn magazines and movies so often feature women touching, kissing, and loving each other. By the way, many women feel a similar, if not as strong fascination towards male homosexuality.

My lover has a huge porn collection in his bedroom: sex magazines, erotic pictures, books, videos and DVDs. When I asked him what he needs all that stuff for, he said that it makes his sex life more exciting. I don't think so at all, I find it much more enjoyable to have a romantic night and make love by candlelight than romping along to a stupid sex movie. But he seems to be addicted to his porn; he doesn't even try to spend a night without it.

Get your lover out of reach of his porn collection by spending a night somewhere else. Tell him how you feel about his attraction to pornographic material, and how much it turns you off. If you love each other, try to work out a compromise. You could let him have his way now and then, if in return he promises to fulfil your wish of spending romantic porn-free nights as well.

I haven't been with a woman for more than ten years. To find sexual relief I masturbate, often three or four times per day. To get into the mood I look at porn magazines. The problem is that it doesn't really satisfy me anymore. As a result I masturbate even more, and that seems to make things worse. I tried to quit the porn magazines, but without them I can't get an erection anymore. Have I become addicted?

You have been masturbating over porn magazines for so long that you have become fixated on this method of finding relief. To sort this out, don't look at porn at all for a week, and don't masturbate during this time.

Every girlfriend I have had so far left me after only a short while for the reason that I want too much sex. I can't help it: I am horny all the time, and I want to try out everything. I love to watch porn films and replay scenes. I have a huge collection of sex toys and other erotic equipment I can spoil a woman with. What I can't understand is why women keep running away from me.

The answer to your question is quite simple: You seem to be obsessed with sex, which is enough to frighten off any female in her right mind. A woman wants to be loved and desired for her personal qualities, and not for her qualifying as a sex object you can try out your sex toys with. If you want to be more successful with women in future, show them more respect, and realise that their needs and wishes are as important as your own.

My fiancé is mad about porn. He tries to hide them, but I find pornographic magazines and videos in his dresser and other places all the time. When I confronted him, he denied being a porn addict. How can I make him realise that he has a serious problem?

You better stop spying on your fiancé. Invading his privacy like that puts your relationship at risk. Young men are normally much more interested in all kinds of sexual matters than young women. There is no harm in that. As long as your fiancé doesn't neglect you, let him have his sex magazines and videos.

Being single, I always watch porn to turn me on when I masturbate. First, I only used to look at nude pictures of lovely women now and then, while now it has to be something stronger, like a porn video. Although it always leaves me with a sort of stale feeling, I can't stop myself from doing it. It has become a bad habit. Do you think I am sick, or even an addict?

I don't think you are sick or an addict. Being single, you depend mainly on yourself and your fantasy to satisfy your sexual needs. There is no harm in stimulating your fantasy with erotic pictures or videos. Just try to do it less often. Overdoing something normally spoils it for you, as you are experiencing right now.

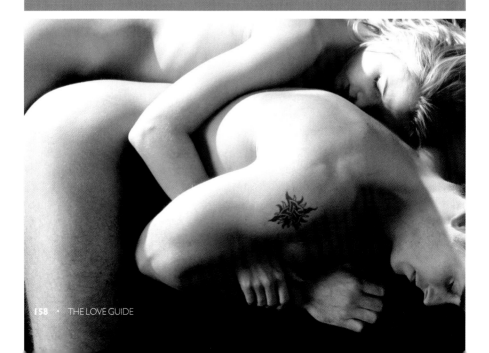

16 Sex Games

The best approach to sex is to view it in a playful manner, as it combines both our intrinsic need to love and our need to play. Unfortunately, this playful instinct often gets lost and the serious facts of life take over which makes it even more important that we remind ourselves that it's normal and healthy to play, especially in bed.

A playful attitude towards sex guarantees more fun, and therefore more satisfaction. So to explore new grounds and keep your sex life exciting keep playing in bed.

Ireland's Favourite Erotic Games

Sex under water is the most popular erotic game in Ireland. Almost every second Irish couple (46%) has made love in the bathtub, under the shower, in the sea –

wherever there's enough water to add to their enjoyment. Almost as many couples (43%) indulge in erotic massage: making it Irish people's second most favoured sex game. For women, an erotic massage doesn't even need to get near the most private parts of their bodies, while men prefer a tender massage of their genitals, above anything else. That's no big surprise I guess, but it's still interesting to see what exactly men and women enjoy most. The third most favourite sex game is mutual masturbation (32%), followed closely by intermammal sex (the rubbing of the penis between the breasts). Sex in public places (29%) comes in fifth place, closely followed by food games (25%) and sex in front of a mirror (24%).

So let's have a more detailed look at our favourite sex games, and check out the kinkier stuff as well.

Sex Under Water

Sex under water is one of the few sex games women are as mad about as men. When you're making love in the sea, a lake, or even a huge whirlpool or hot tub, you manage positions you can only dream about under the normal laws of gravity. The best place for underwater sex games is the sea. Intruders can only see clearly what

you do above the water line, while what you are up to underneath remains a mystery. The odd snorkeller might catch a glimpse of your sex game, but that only adds to the kicks underwater sex has to offer.

Sex in the tub isn't too bad either. If you don't have a hot tub, a bathtub will do. Most bathtubs are a tight fit, but with a healthy resourceful attitude you will still find the right position to make love. Try this position: the man can stretch out in the tub while his lover kneels above him. If you don't mind a good bit of water splashing over the rim, she can stretch out on the opposite side of the tub, joining him in the middle.

If you haven't got a bathtub then try it in the shower. You can make love from behind standing up, with her bending over slightly while he holds on to her hips. But the best sex you are ever going to get under the shower is oral sex. Soap each other off from top to toe, then after rinsing off well, get a taste of each other's genitals. This love game is ideal to introduce your lover to oral sex, as it alleviates any worries about hygiene.

'Love in the water is the best,' says Sarah (23) from Co. Dublin. 'I can't wait for our next holidays. Last year in Cyprus, we kept seeking out deserted beaches,

...nd made love there in the sea. Now we have to make do with the bathtub. It's a bit too cramped for my taste, but at least I can feel the water on my skin while we make love.'

Erotic Massage

Erotic massage is usually a woman's domain. Women mainly massage their men for two reasons: the hope of getting a good massage themselves, and the second is the assumption that their lover enjoys the same pleasures as they do. Normally, couples work this misunderstanding out quickly, and then find a compromise that is extremely satisfying for both parties. While he concentrates for a long time on her back, buttocks, inner thighs and breasts before moving to her private parts, she doesn't spend too much time massaging other parts of his body but starts working on his genital area more or less straight away.

To make an erotic massage even more exotic, apply scented oil onto your bodies, and then gently rub it in to make your skin more sensitive.

Mutual Masturbation

Maybe this sex game sounds a bit boring, but it can be very exciting under the right circumstances and in the right place. You can masturbate each other relatively discreetly in places that don't allow you to do more if you don't want to get arrested for indecent behaviour. Or you can do it in your bedroom, just for a change of routine. Apply a lube to make your touch feel different. Combine mutual masturbation with dirty talk to add to the excitement. Fantasise about all the other erotic things you want to try out with each other.

To make mutual masturbation more exciting, watch your partner's face while you touch each other.

Cleavage Sex – Sex Between the Breasts

Every third Irish couple (34%) practices cleavage sex or to give it its scientific name intermammae sex – the caressing and rubbing of the penis between the breasts. It's one of the trickier games, and not easy to manage, especially when her breasts aren't that big. If her breasts are small, it's best if she sits on top of him, bending forward to let her breasts dangle above his pelvis. He can then carefully press them inward to let them engulf his penis. Another technique is if she lies down on her back, pressing her breasts up from both sides, while he moves in between them, kneeling above her.

Sex in Public Places

There are many public places that couples use for their love games. We are not talking about discreet places like a deserted beach, a woodshed in the middle of nowhere or even a lovers' lane. It is the really exposed public places that these couples play their games in: highly frequented parks, pubs, theatres, escalators, car parks, even taxis. The special kick is the risk of getting caught anytime.

Evelyn (24) and her boyfriend are almost obsessed by adding new places to their list. 'The craziest thing we've done so far was a quickie in the loo. Although people must have heard us, nobody bothered to disturb us. The reaction we got were a few broad grins when we finally came out.'

If sex outside turns you on, bear in mind that people who happen to stumble across you might feel offended.

Food Games

Sex games involving food have become very popular, especially after the infamous scene from the film 9$\frac{1}{2}$ weeks. It has become more and more popular to dish up little treats on your own body and to have your partner eat or lick them off. Those games involve anything from fruit, cream, ice cream to soft cheese, pâté, sausages, and whatever else you can imagine.

There are basically three variations of this game. The first and most innocent one is to just dine off your partner's belly and breast. The

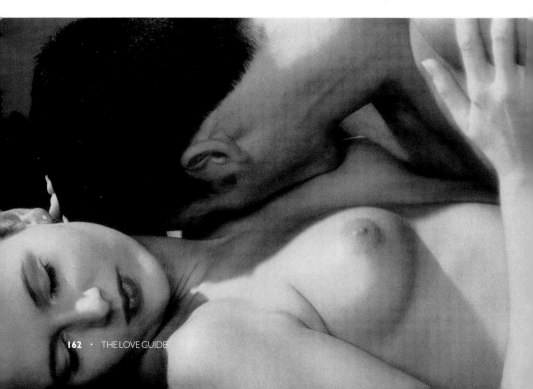

second most popular is to apply some delicious treat onto his penis. Some guys use honey, others choose chocolate cream, some go for stronger stuff, like paté or cream cheese or whatever else they find in the fridge.

'My fiancé once wanted oral sex, but was too shy to ask for it. So after dinner, he asked whether we could have dessert in bed. He'd bought some fresh strawberries, and whipped up lots of cream. When I came out of the bathroom after my shower, I found him propped up in bed, with a line of strawberries leading down from his breastbone to the tip of his penis. Every strawberry was tipped with some whipped cream, and so was the tip of his penis. He got what he wanted that night, without even asking...', reveals Nicole (23) from Co. Meath.

The third and most intimate game is when a woman hides treats for her lover to find at the entrance of her vagina.

'This game is one of my favourites, it never fails to arouse my man's sexual appetite,' admits Natasha (28). 'I have tried out everything from chocolate bars, to sausages and bananas. And he always goes for the treat.'

Sex in Front of a Mirror

Almost a quarter of all Irish couples (24%) have tried out this sexy game: making love in front of a mirror. It is hard enough to watch your partner while you're making love, and you never get a full picture of the two of you together – except when you are in front of a mirror. To watch both of you in ecstasy together is a real turn on. It's much better than watching love scenes in a film, or watching porn, because it's reality. You can see what you are doing, and feel what you see, and that's hard to beat.

To get the best out if it, try out different positions in front of a mirror. Some positions even allow you to watch the most intimate details of your lovemaking. Like the pressed position, where she lies on her back with her legs pulled up and her feet pressing against his chest, while he kneels in front of her.

Vibrator Games

More than one out of every five Irish couples (22%) plays vibrator games. Vibrators are mainly, but not solely, used during foreplay. Sometimes they are used for teasing games all over the body, but their main job is without a doubt to stimulate the clitoris. Many men find it difficult to arouse their partner by just using their hands. The vibrator is a helpful tool: move it lightly around the clitoris, and it sends shivers up a girl's spine. It can be inserted as well, although most men prefer to keep the privilege of getting inside there for themselves.

While these humming sex toys serve mainly to please a woman, some are especially designed to suit a man as well.

'My guy loves to feel something up his bum when we have sex. I used to stimulate him with my finger, but then I got him an anal stimulator as a surprise for his birthday. It is much smaller than the vibrator I have for myself, but it's definitely doing a great job. My boyfriend absolutely loves the feeling, and I could swear that he comes much stronger when I use it on him.' Aine (31) from Co. Dublin.

Shaving Pubic Hair

Some men regard it as a big turn on to shave their lover 'down there'. This wish is simple to explain: they want to see those most intimate parts completely naked, to explore and caress them. It also feels so much better to make love without having to fight your way through a jungle of pubic hair, especially if you are into some intimate kissing.

An intimate shave is normally followed by the man doing a close check-up, so it's worth letting him have a go. There is no harm in trying this out. In case you are wondering – your pubic hair will grow back. You might feel a bit itchy for a couple of days with newly grown stubble, but then it will grow back as per normal.

In case you girls fancy shaving your lover – men are very reluctant to try it out, as dense pubic hair is one of the signs that prove their masculinity.

'I love to shave my lover,' explains Eamon (28), 'when she first allowed me to give her a wet shave it was the sexiest experience I've ever had. But then she insisted that I let her shave me as well. I didn't like the idea at all, but I couldn't say no. So she had a go at it. I still think I looked stupid being all naked down there, I was reminded of my early teens when I couldn't wait to grow some body hair to look like a man. But my girlfriend loved it, she says my penis looks even bigger when I'm shaved.'

Sipping Champagne from the Belly Button

This sex game is most popular among young couples. Although it is without doubt arousing to feel the champagne bubble in such a sensitive spot, the game is not so much about sipping from the belly button itself, but more about tracing and licking up all the precious drops and rivulets that get spilled.

It's a great game to carefully introduce a woman to the pleasures of oral sex, for you can be sure that at least some drops of champagne will find their way to the genitals, where of course they need to be licked off.

Striptease

Striptease has become an increasingly popular sex game, with recent films feeding the trend. You have to dress sexy, and then spoil your partner with an erotic, exotic dance, slowly shedding your clothes, piece by piece. It is important to pick the right music, outfit and special sexy underwear. Then practise in front of a mirror to make sure that your performance has the effect you wish for.

A well-performed striptease is a perfect start to an erotic night. Striptease is no longer just a female domain – men are catching up, inspired by films, video clips, and male stripper groups. Most women absolutely love dancing, and they love the sight of a masculine body. To see both combined in an erotic dance, even if it's far from being professional, is a huge turn on.

If you want your striptease to succeed first of all you need an erotic outfit that comes off easily while you're dancing. For your own sake, don't wear the comfortable old briefs or underwear that your mum got you. Check out a fashion magazine to see what's chic at the moment. Then either go for it, or scout the shops for something exclusive that you feel more comfortable with.

Then, you need to pick a piece of music that allows you to shed your clothes, piece by piece, at a leisurely pace. To get your movements and expression right, practise in front of a mirror before you give your first performance – to make sure that your striptease is going to be a triumph.

Sex Talk on the Internet

With more and more computers around, there's an increase in the number of complete strangers joining chat rooms to exchange interests and to talk dirty to each other. One of the greatest kicks is anonymity. You can pretend to be whoever you wish to be, give yourself a fancy name, and then chat away anonymously, laying open your kinkiest fantasies and desires. And there are hardly any taboos in chat rooms; you can have a chat about almost everything, whether it's normal stuff like making love from behind or unusual wishes like wearing latex, fancying nappies or playing outlandish games.

While most participants hide behind false identities during an erotic net chat, some build up serious relationships, and even go so far as to meet their partner in person. Some people who met in chat rooms have even ended up getting married.

'I met my current girlfriend in an Internet chat room,' describes Tom (43) from Co. Cork. 'We have the same fantasies, and found out after a few weeks that we were getting really curious about each other. At that stage we were still using our code names. Then we sent each other pictures, and shortly after that we met for the first time. We spent a fabulous weekend together, living out all our fantasies. At the moment we are looking for a place to move in together.'

To be on the safe side be careful when arranging to meet someone you have chatted to on the Internet. It's a good idea to meet in a public place first and not to give out any personal details like your address or phone number before you meet up.

Sexy Photos

Taking sexy photos has become very popular since digital technology allows couples to enjoy their private sex photos without the embarrassing visit to a photo shop.

Filming sex games has become another favourite with more and more couples using digital video cameras. While most couples film their home sex movies themselves, the more adventurous ones team up with a like-minded couple to take turns filming and acting.

'We are an open-minded group of three couples,' tells Eliza (43) from Co. Wexford. 'We meet to swap partners and have fun. Filming each other is our newest game. Then one of us takes the camera home, and puts an erotic film together, which we watch as a start up at our next meeting. It is great to lean back on your couch, and watch yourself on television like you were a porn star.'

Playing Erotic Film Scenes

Young people especially enjoy re-enacting erotic scenes they've seen in films. As you slip into playing a role it is much easier to become bolder and to overcome old inhibitions. After all, you are only play acting and somebody else has written the script.

'My husband and I often pick out sex scenes from films, then pretend to be those famous stars, and replay their sex-scenes in our bedroom. Only we don't stop when it gets too hot for the screen, but play on and on, bringing the scene to its end,' says Ita (22) from Co. Dublin.

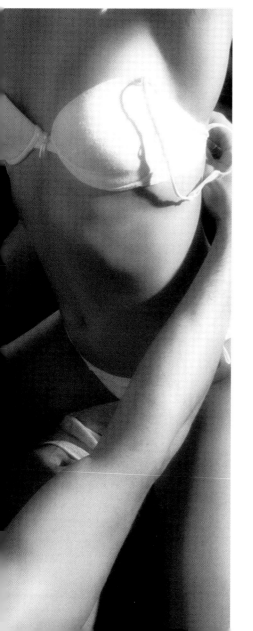

Other Sex Games

There are many other sex games that are less popular, but just as exciting. Some couples love role-playing — she pretends to be his housemaid, he pretends to be her callboy — there are lots of enticing variations. The idea behind role-playing is to evoke and live out fantasies. Many roles that couples slip into involve a difference in authority levels — like boss/secretary, teacher/student, or in its extreme master/slave.

Another sex game is axillary inter-course, where the man rubs his penis under his lover's armpit.

Other couples play on the strange side, enjoying games that most people would never dream of playing, enjoying Golden Showers and more. But then as long as you are grown-ups, and both enjoy what you are doing, there is no harm in experimenting. Although, there is one sex game that you should stay clear of — autoerotic asphyxiation. It means masturbating while you deprive yourself of oxygen by self-strangulation, for example by hanging, to increase sexual pleasure. This game is incredibly dangerous, and leads to many involuntary deaths. It is especially dangerous in combination with self-bondage.

Ireland's Top Erotic Games

The answers to the multiple-choice survey question, 'What are your favourite erotic games?' were as follows:

Sex Under Water	46%
Erotic Massage	43%
Mutual Masturbation	32%
Cleavage Sex	31%
Sex in Public Places	29%
Food Games	25%
Sex in Front of a Mirror	24%
Vibrator Games	22%
Shaving Pubic Hair	21%
Sipping Champagne from the Belly Button	18%
Striptease	15%
Sex Talk on the Internet	9%
Sexy Photos	8%
Playing Erotic Film Scenes	7%

TIPS

Keep your love life alive by experimenting.

Try out new sex games.

Remember you have the best chance of a happy love life if you approach sex with a playful attitude.

Sex Dictionary

AUTOEROTIC ASPHYXIATION
The practise of masturbating while you deprive yourself of oxygen by self-strangulation to increase sexual pleasure. Extremely dangerous, and has led to many involuntary deaths every year.

AXILLARY INTERCOURSE
Rubbing of penis in the partner's armpit.

CLEAVAGE SEX
Clevage sex is rubbing the penis between a woman's breasts. Also called 'Spanish' or intermammae.

GOLDEN SHOWERS
Urinating on a sexual partner for stimulation.

SEXUAL ROLE-PLAYING
Playing a role while you have sex to live out a fantasy.

Q&A

We have tried sex between my breasts, but didn't really succeed. The only way we managed was by me holding my breasts up and squeezing them together the whole time, while he rubbed himself between them, but that's sort of awkward for me. Is there a better way of doing it?

You can wear a tight bra to push your breasts up and squeeze them together, that's less tiresome than holding them in place with your hands. And a sexy bra definitely adds to the excitement of this love game, even if it restricts your choice of positions.

We used to enjoy making love standing up, facing a mirror. I lifted my wife (nine stone) onto my penis. It was so arousing to move her up and down. Recently my strength has decreased, so we had to give it up. I'm 50; do you think I'm too old for sex games like this?

You are not too old. Strong-men of your age group can easily lift much more than nine stone. Weight lifting will help you to lift your wife again. Join a gym to build up your muscles, or get some dumbbells to exercise at home. Or try out other positions in front of the mirror. If you like it standing up, lift one of your wife's legs over your hips to make love. This position allows you a perfect view of the intimate details of your lovemaking.

I fantasise about wearing nappies, wetting myself, and then having a strict nanny first punish, then change me. I realize that it would be hard to find a woman who would be willing to play along, but would you say its okay for me to at least wear nappies on my own, and where could I find some?

Try not to get fixated on such an unusual sexual dream as wearing nappies. It is almost impossible to find a woman who will play along, so you won't be fully satisfied when you live out your fantasy, but will only find yourself longing for more. If you want to try it out anyway, you can get nappies for grown ups in a pharmacy.

I am never really relaxed when we make love. Could an erotic massage help me to relax and get into the right mood?

Erotic massage with your partner is definitely worth a try, as it will help you to relax, and turn you on as well. Buy an illustrated book that shows techniques and positions, and some scented massage oil. You can easily find all you need on the Internet: explanations of how erotic massage works, experiences of couples who've tried it, and offers on books, oils, scents and much more. Use a search engine to look for the right keywords, and you'll get a list of Internet pages on the subject.

I would love to bathe in champagne, like the stars do. But surely it's a waste to let the expensive stuff run down the drain. What do you think?

If it's not one of your life's dearest dreams, forget about it. A bath in champagne is pretty cold, and the stuff feels rather sticky. The only pleasant aspect is the tickling sensation the champagne bubbles leave on your skin, and you can enjoy that feeling much better in a whirlpool. It takes at least 150 bottles of champagne to fill a bath – costing you a small fortune. So I think you're much better off just sipping the odd glass of champagne comfortably whilst sitting in a whirlpool. To feel it on your skin, pour some over your breasts and belly, or any other place you fancy.

I want to film our lovemaking, but my girlfriend is completely against it. I can't understand why she is so prudish. How can I persuade her to play along?

It's not prudish to refuse to act in a homemade porn video. There is always the risk that others might see your little masterpiece, and that would be extremely embarrassing for your girlfriend. If you want her to play along, respect her privacy. Your best chance of her fulfilling your wish is if you promise her that she can keep the only copy of this very intimate film.

My boyfriend wants me to shave my pubic hair but I don't want to look like a little girl down there. How can I talk him out of it?

Try to 'convince' him with a deal: tell him you are going to shave your pubic hair if he does the same. That should make him see your point. It's hard to imagine him wanting to look like a little boy. I bet he'll back out of the deal.

My wife has found out that I chat with other ladies on the Internet. She feels betrayed, while I'm only having a harmless bit of fun. What's your opinion – is it cheating to chat online?

Chatting online is a harmless way of cheating. I'm sure you wouldn't be too pleased yourself if you'd found out your own wife was chatting on the net with other guys so try to understand her reaction. Explain to her that you see it as a harmless game. If your wife insists that it's cheating to chat online, but you don't want to give it up, invite her along to participate in your sex chat on the net. More and more couples spice up their sex life by chatting anonymously with kindred spirits.

Does golden showers mean bathing in champagne?

No, this term is a bit misleading, as it makes you think of something special and precious while in fact it's a glamorous term for a rude sexual practice. It's not about bathing in champagne, but about peeing on each other.

We feel we are too young to have intercourse, but we both like masturbating. Would it be weird if we masturbate together?

It is not weird at all if you masturbate together, on the contrary, touching yourselves and each other is a great way for the two of you to explore your sexuality. Many teenagers rush into sexual adventures that they are much too young for, like having intercourse. Rushing things means spoiling the experience. You are doing the right thing by progressing step by step, and at your own pace.

I like to feel a rubber penis up my bum when I sleep with my wife, it makes me get a firmer erection, and I come stronger. Is it safe, or could I become gay?

You don't become gay from using a rubber penis. The anus is a very sensitive area, and many heterosexual men like to have it stimulated, as do some women as well. To avoid doing any damage by playing with a rubber penis, use a small one, apply lots of lubrication, and stop when you feel uncomfortable.

My boyfriend seems to have lost interest in me; he hardly ever makes a move anymore to make love to me. He prefers to watch TV. What do you think, could I lure him into bed with a striptease?

I am sure that a sexy outfit and a striptease would do the trick of getting your boyfriend into bed. Try it some night when he is not watching his favourite programme or an 'important' match. You should also talk to your boyfriend about his apparent disinterest in making love to find out whether something's wrong with your relationship from his point of view.

We would love to try out cleavage sex, but my breasts are below average in size, they become almost invisible when I lie down on my back. Is there a better position?

Let your lover lie down on his back, and then kneel over him. Place his penis between your dangling breasts, then press them together with your hands to firmly encircle him. As a special kick, place a pillow under his head, so that he can watch himself making love to your breasts.

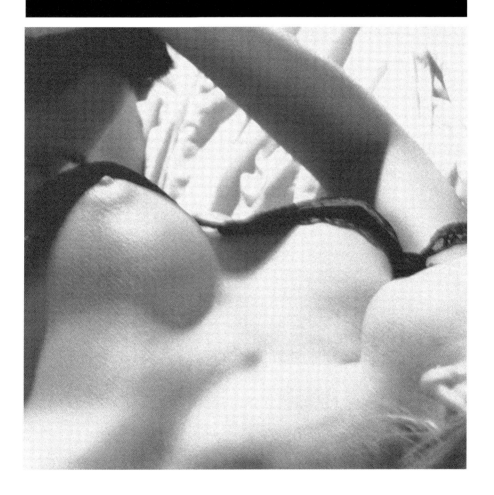

17 Sex Toys

Not so long ago sex toys were still unavailable on the Irish market. Vibrators, fun condoms, blow-up dolls and other erotic items were only brought in as exotic souvenirs from holidays abroad.

Then the silent invasion began. A vibrator from a weekend in Amsterdam, a pouting blow-up doll from one of the numerous sex shops in Hamburg St. Pauli, then the first adult shop arrived in Ireland. And now, especially thanks to the Internet, you can buy whatever you fancy.

'It's great that you can do your sex toy shopping on the Internet, although I miss the atmosphere of the real shop, where you can touch everything and compare. I still go on those shopping trips with my friends. Last time we bought presents for our boyfriends, phosphorescent condoms in eerie colours that light in the dark. And for my mom I bought a vibrator that is disguised as a lipstick. She'll crack up when she sees it,' reveals Monica (23).

The variety of sex toys on the market is amazing. It would take you days to scout out the wide range of vibrators and dildos alone. There is hardly a toy that can't be bought. There are even ones that you can heat up in the microwave for added comfort. It's not only the classic sex toys that are flying off the shelves, more advanced and unusual stuff is also selling well. Let's have a look at what's available.

Vibrators

Vibrators have the reputation of being joysticks for lonely hearts, but that's doing them an injustice. They are far more than that. Our survey revealed that one out of every four Irish women uses a vibrator, and the trend is rising, with sex toys now easily available here. Not only singles enjoy vibrators, but more and more married women as well. So these humming toys add lots of pleasure not only to the sex life of single women but to that of millions of couples as well. Couples use vibrators mainly during foreplay.

'First I was reluctant,' admits Bob (47) from Co. Dublin, 'but the vibrator takes a lot of pressure off me. It definitely helps my wife to get an orgasm. It was almost impossible before. Now I tease her with the vibrator during foreplay. When I make love to her afterwards, she comes within a few minutes.'

Men can't help but wonder why a woman would prefer an artificial penis rather than having a real and eager one. The answer is simple: a vibrator almost never fails to produce an orgasm. Part of the reason is that a woman can control the type, and pace, of stimulation herself. It's up to her whether she holds it against her clitoris, or lets it slip into the vagina to do its miraculous work there.

Another plus: a vibrator never sweats, never argues, and is always willing to perform according to your wishes, and always there when you need it. Most models fit easily into every handbag. Their main flaw is that you have to replace their batteries every so often, so might end up having to operate your sex toy manually.

Different Types

Let's look at the different types available and discover that vibrators are much more than a mere substitute for 'the real thing'.

Vibrators come in dozens of different shapes, colours and models. The classic one is basically a rubber replica of a real penis, designed with a lot of attention to detail. Some models come with scrotum included for an even more realistic feel. Others have flapping, so called 'rabbit ears', at their base, to stimulate the clitoris.

The range starts from a simple one-speed model to a fully adjustable and purely high-tech specimen. Newer ones can be worked with a remote control, and special models spoil the customer with a humming rotation head. Waterproof models are specially designed for pleasure in the shower or bathtub. Other models will take any kind of fluid that can be used later to simulate ejaculation.

You can even buy a vibrator that can be heated up to body temperature in the microwave. Another special treat is the extremely flexible dual-action, double-vibrator with two heads – one on each end. The so called G-spot vibrator, easily recognisable by its unnatural looking inward facing bend, promises to massage the often described, but still not agreed on G-spot, inside the vagina.

The material vibrators are made from ranges from soft vinyl to hard metal. Some vibrators are made of a hard jelly-like material, others have a special coating that makes them sparkle or glow in the dark. The colour range is amazing as well – all colours of the rainbow are catered for. Their size ranges from a couple of inches to intimidating 15-inch-giants. Vibrators even come in disguise. The lipstick-shaped vibrator is almost a classic by now. Another clever model is the small toy you can discreetly put on your key chain.

'I have tried out many of the new models,' admits Hettie (48) from Co. Laois, 'but my favourite is still the old fashioned penis shaped one in a natural colour. I have even tried a microwavable one, but instead of heating it up in the kitchen, I'd rather hold an old fashioned model against my belly for a few minutes to get it to the right temperature.'

Dildos

Dildos are a much simpler design than vibrators. They look more or less like a real penis and, as they don't have batteries, can only be operated manually. They don't vibrate but their silence ensures more discretion. While they miss the vibration sensation, they won't give you away by humming, if you need to be discreet.

You can also find strap-on dildos. There are two types of strap-on dildos available – one that is held by a band around your loins and the other is built into a more solid harness you wear around your hips.

Strap-on Dildos

There's a great selection of strap-on products on the market, for men and women, as well. Basically, a dildo is attached to a harness to allow the person wearing it to penetrate somebody else.

Special luxurious models come with penis rings attached. Another fascinating specimen has a multi-speed vibrating egg for self-stimulation embedded in the panty. There're also double strap-on dildos that allow vaginal and anal stimulation simultaneously. Another type has a built in anal plug. Some models are hollow to accommodate a penis inside them, while others are solid.

Strap-on dildos are mainly used by men who suffer from potency problems, or by guys who dream of having a bigger penis.

Special Condoms

Special condoms are much more than mere contraceptives. Fitted out with a special surface and coating, they can intensify sexual pleasure. One out of every four Irish couples (27%), enjoy their benefits. There is a vast range out there, for almost every taste: super glide coatings, special tastes like banana, tops in the shape of a devil, surfaces spiced up with rings of soft beads or creepy looking spikes, and much more. The luminous condom is still an old favourite. This old-timer looks inconspicuous as long as the light is on, but starts glowing as soon as it gets dark.

Penis Rings

Years ago, penis rings were merely what their name implies – simple rings that slipped over the penis to keep the blood in, to maintain and prolong an erection, and at the same time mechanically rub against the clitoris. Their main purpose is still the same, but they are much more sophisticated. The contemporary penis ring is made of soft material, vibrates, and, if you are willing to pay the price, can be mastered by remote control.

'It is just a change of our daily routine,' explains Betty (32) from Co. Dublin. 'We sometimes use sex toys just to try out something new. After all, you don't want to miss out on anything. The penis ring was fun for a while, but the tickle of the new was soon over.'

Pocket Pussies and Penises

You might find it too awkward to handle a life-sized love doll, or find it difficult to store it. A more convenient and compact sex toy is a replica of only the male or female genitals.

There are fake vaginas for sale, as well as very realistic looking female buttocks with anus and vagina. Some of the most popular ones on the market are replicas of famous porn stars' bits and pieces. On the package you even get a picture of the real genitals for comparison.

You can find penis replicas as well, which are very solid and realistic looking. And they promise to last most endurance tests.

Bonds and Handcuffs

One out of every seven Irish couples plays games of bondage, using everything from soft scarves to chains and handcuffs to playfully tie their partner up for sex. The main method is tying your partner's wrists to the bedposts or the head of the bed, or using shackles to bind their wrists or ankles together.

Couples normally use bonds in a playful way, giving each other the chance to end the game and get away at any time.

'I love it when my wife shackles my wrists to the bedposts and then gets on top of me to take me. She is fully in charge then, which is a big turn on,' explains Richard from Co. Kildare. 'The flimsy handcuffs she got in a sex shop couldn't hold me for a second, but nonetheless it's extremely sexy to be at her mercy.'

Some bondage fans take the game much more seriously, getting an erotic

Love Dolls

One out of every 16 Irish men (6%) has had a sexual encounter with an inflatable rubber doll. Love dolls (or blow-up dolls) have so far – no big surprise – almost exclusively been used by lonely men.

The basic models are cheap crude balloons that roughly resemble a female form. The expensive models are a bit more exotic and detailed, with real hair, real-feel breasts, and a vibrating vagina. Some models come with a remote control.

There is a doll for every taste: whether it's the tarty blow-up doll, or the sensitive sucking one, with a vibrating mouth. The hygiene enthusiast can even get them with a removable vagina for easier cleaning. The enhanced models come with a repair kit in case you flatten them.

Of course the days are over when only female rubber dolls were available. Nowadays inflatable male rubber dolls are also available, life-sized and with all the necessary anatomical equipment. It goes without saying that these are available in different sizes and colours, with a vibrating penis and a tight anus if preferred.

You can even purchase a doll with both penis and breasts. The penis vibrates on request, while the breasts feel as close to real ones as possible.

kick out of restraining their partner's bodily movements, using collars, harnesses, chains, padlocks, and innumerable other devices. Have a look at the BDSM chapter to find out more details about this.

Whatever you are getting up to special care must be taken during games of bondage to ensure that neither you nor your partner gets hurt.

Ecstasy Balls

Ecstasy balls are one of the classic sex toys. Also called love balls or Japanese geisha balls. They are made up of two or more beads on a string, often filled with multiple smaller beads that roll around in the outer ones. Modern ones come with a built in vibrator, even with a remote control, while older and plainer versions only work mechanically. When they are pushed into the vagina, ecstasy balls usually fulfil what their name promises – ecstasy.

The original ecstasy balls came from the Far East, where Japanese geishas used them to train their vaginal muscles. Geisha balls still fulfil that purpose, more or less all over the world now. On average, eight per cent of all women use them.

Ecstasy balls aren't just restricted to the privacy of a bedroom – they can be worn everywhere and at any time. You can even leave them in all day, now and then.

'I have always been kind of old fashioned,' admits Maura (30) from Co. Dublin. 'But then I got those ecstasy balls for my thirtieth birthday. I was dumbstruck at first, so I put the present aside, but then tried it out later. I now often wear the geisha balls during the day. It is nice to feel them moving inside me, and they are tiny enough to feel comfortable whatever I'm doing.'

Anal Stimulators

Anal stimulators are sex toys especially designed for anal stimulation. They're anal beads, not dissimilar to geisha balls, which are placed in the anus and then pulled out for stimulation. Some beads come with vibrating balls, which promise an extra intense feeling.

Butt plugs, in different forms and shapes, for prostate massage and anal masturbation are also available, as well as anal vibrators. There's a variety of anal lubes and condoms to keep anal games comfortable and safe.

Others

The list of available sex toys is getting longer and longer and the variety has become more extensive. You can get pocket masturbators, oral sex simulators, penis sleeves and penis extensions, any toy you could wish for. Toys for fun, and toys that might help you to have a more fulfilling sex life.

So if you are curious, there is no harm in checking out what's on the market. You don't have to buy or try out anything, but it can't hurt to know what is available. You never know, by checking out what's new you might stumble over the sex toy that will fulfil your wildest dreams. Take your partner along for a bit of an adventure.

Party Toys

If you are organising a stag or a hen party, a party kit containing a wild and wide range of sex toys, especially designed as party gags and presents will get you started. For more fun toys you can get penis and bum shaped candles and edible treats.

If you don't have anyone to go to a party with you can get an inflatable guy or girl to accompany you. They won't look too offensive, as they are just balloons, lacking any cavities for penetration. Or, if you don't mind looking ridiculous, for a laugh you could get a set of pecker glasses, with penis attached.

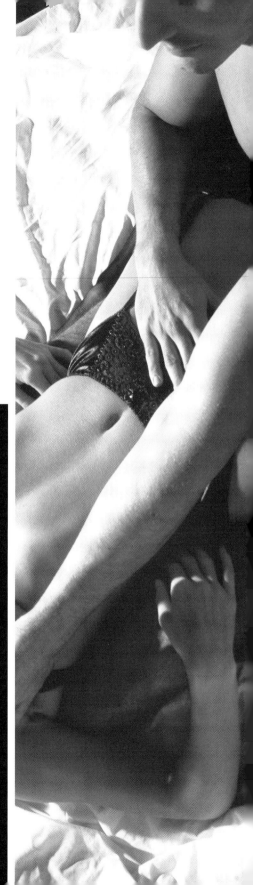

TIPS

The Merits of Vibrators:
Stimulating during foreplay
Consoling in lonely moments

A temporary alternative for
single women.

Sex Dictionary

ANAL BEADS
Beads or small balls on a string that can be inserted into the anus to then be pulled out for sexual stimulation.

BUTT PLUG
A device that is inserted into the anus. It often has a flat base to prevent it from disappearing into the body.

CLITORAL STIMULATOR
A normal vibrating device that is worn inside underwear, or can be attached to the clitoris with straps.

DILDO
A fake penis, mainly made of plastic.

DOUBLE DILDO
A dildo with two heads that can be enjoyed by two people at the same time.

ECSTASY BALLS
Balls or beads on a string that can be inserted into the vagina for sexual stimulation. Also called geisha balls.

LOVE DOLL
Inflatable human shaped rubber dolls with mouth, vagina, and anus to allow penetration.

PENIS EXTENSION
A partially hollow dildo like device that can be slipped over the penis to extend its length.

PENIS RING
A sex toy that is slipped over the penis to keep the blood in to ensure a firm erection and to stimulate the clitoris.

POCKET PUSSY
Shaped like vagina with a hole to allow penetration.

SEX TOY
Objects like vibrators or sex dolls, designed to give sexual pleasure.

STRAP-ON
A penis shaped object that is built into a harness, and can be worn strapped around the hips or pelvis.

VIBRATOR
A vibrating electric penis shaped sex toy. The wide range runs from vibrating fake lipsticks to precise imitations of a man's penis.

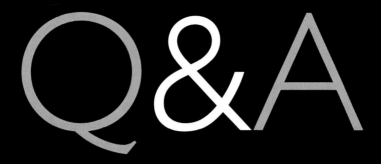

I had never had an orgasm when I slept with a man, until I started to wear ecstasy balls. Now I orgasm regularly, but I worry whether there might be any long-term effects. Could I get frigid from wearing ecstasy balls all the time?

My husband can't satisfy me in bed. The only time that I have an orgasm is when I help myself while he sleeps with me. The few times he tried to arouse me with his hands were a disaster. I want him to use a vibrator to turn me on, but I'm terrified to ask him.

You have to talk to your husband frankly. If he can't arouse you, the two of you obviously have to do something about it. Before you confront him with a sex toy, show him how to stimulate you with his hands and lips. If that doesn't work out, tell him about your idea of getting a vibrator. He might be reluctant at first, but will enjoy it after a while, especially when he sees that it is working out for you.

I want to buy a vibrator. I would also like to see the whole range of sex toys that are on offer nowadays. Can I visit a sex shop on my own? Or would people make fun of me because I'm a woman on my own?

Of course you can visit an adult shop on your own. The other shoppers are there for the same reason as you are, so why would they make fun of you? And the folks working in a sex shop won't give you a second glance either. After all, an adult shop isn't anything else but a normal retail business like so many others.

Getting older, I find it much harder to find a woman to share a cosy night with. More bluntly, there isn't much I can do to satisfy my sexual needs. Women at least have their vibrators – but what about us men? I don't think there's anything comparable for us. Are there any sex toys for men at all?

The sex-toy industry mainly aims at men, not women. Correspondingly, there are lots of toys to fulfil a single man's sexual needs. In adult shops and on the Internet you can find a wide range of masturbation aids, fake latex vaginas, life-size inflatable sex-dolls and many more.

My best friend is crazy about her vibrator. Ever since she got this sex toy, you always see a happy smile on her face. She says it is much better than having a man. I would like to try one out myself, but I'm afraid that it might not be safe. As far as I know vibrators work with batteries. Isn't that dangerous?

I have never heard of anybody who seriously hurt herself using a vibrator. If you feel uneasy about electric vibrators, use a dildo without batteries. There is such a wide range of different models on the market that I am sure you will find one that suits you. I doubt that using a vibrator beats being with a man, but give it a try and find out for yourself.

I am on the lookout for a new partner, but it might take a while until I find somebody. So I thought that it might be a good idea to get myself a vibrator for lonely nights. I have already made inquiries where to find one, but my best friend warned me that I might get hooked on vibrators. Is that true?

It is true that many women enjoy love games with their vibrator so much that they use them regularly, often daily, but I wouldn't call that getting hooked. There is no harm in finding new ways of getting pleasure, and to get satisfied daily. Don't let your best friend's doubts put you off.

My boyfriend went through my stuff and found my vibrator. When he asked me what I needed it for, I made up a lame excuse about the vibrator being there for ages, and that of course I don't use it on myself. He doesn't believe me, and brings this embarrassing topic up again and again. What can I do to stop him?

First of all, tell your boyfriend that he has no right to go through your things. He should respect your privacy. Then let him know the truth about your vibrator. Explain to him why you have it and what it's good for, if he promises in return never to bring that topic up again. If he discovers that you actually use it, it might hurt his male ego, but it will also make him try harder to satisfy you in bed.

Every time I have sex with my inflatable rubber doll, I develop an itchy rash on my penis. Is it possible that I could catch something from the doll, maybe an infection, or even AIDS?

If you don't share your doll with others, and give it a good wash every time you have used it, you won't catch any infection. You probably suffer from a latex allergy. Check exactly what material your doll is made of, and then get an allergy test. If you are indeed allergic, you can get special latex free condoms from a pharmacy.

My mother found my sex doll when she was cleaning up my room. Luckily it was still in its package. I had bought it for myself, but made up a story saying I brought it home from Amsterdam for a friend of mine. I'm terribly frustrated that I can't keep my doll, but it can't be helped. Is there something smaller and easier to hide that could fulfil the same purpose as a sex doll?

Sure, there are smaller sex toys, and ones that are easier to hide, but they probably wouldn't make up for the loss of your sex doll. So why not keep it? Tell your mom that you will clean your room on your own from now on – you should do that anyway. Then get a new wardrobe or maybe a chest that you can lock to guarantee a bit of privacy.

My girlfriend wants me to wear a condom that covers the testicles as well as the penis. I would fulfil her wish, but aren't those things dangerous? And anyway, where would I find them?

You find special condoms like that in adult shops or on the Internet. They aren't dangerous, so there is no harm in trying them out.

My fiancé wants to try out handcuffs. We have tried out games of bondage before, using scarves. I don't feel comfortable with that idea of getting handcuffed at all, but missed the opportunity to tell him from the start. He might bring handcuffs home soon, expecting me to be delighted. How can I get out of this?

Be open with your fiancé. Tell him that it's okay to play bondage games, but that you feel uncomfortable with the idea of using handcuffs. It's important for you to ensure that you can get out of a bondage game anytime, in case it is getting too rough for your taste. So you better stick to soft material. Instead of using handcuffs stick to the harmless games that you have been enjoying so far.

I have heard that wearing a penis ring you get an extra hard erection. Is it harmless to wear such a penis ring, and could I use a simple rubber band instead, as that is much cheaper?

Don't use a rubber band. Think about what you are doing: if you tie a rubber band tight around the base of your penis, you are going to cause a potentially dangerous and painful blood congestion. If you want to try out a penis ring, at least get a decent one from the specialised trade to avoid medical problems.

I have bought myself some Japanese ecstasy balls. When I first tried them, I really loved the feeling – so I left them in. When I checked the next morning, they were gone. Is it possible that they dissolved in my vagina?

You probably took them out and misplaced them. Ecstasy balls can't dissolve. They are made from solid material. If you can't find them, let your gynaecologist have a look to make sure that they didn't get lost inside you.

My girlfriend wants to penetrate my anus with objects, such as pens and drumsticks. She promises to use lubrication and not to push them in too far, but I'm not sure. I don't want to carry out her fetish, but I don't want to let her down either, as she is always open to my ideas.

If you don't want to let your girlfriend down, give it a try, but be very careful with the choice of objects for this sex game. The anus is very sensitive and more vulnerable than a vagina, so you shouldn't allow any objects that are too rigid or have sharp edges. To be on the safe side, you can use an anal stimulator or something that is similar in texture and shape. You might not enjoy it, but at least you needn't be worried about getting hurt.

I have tried out rubber dolls, and have experimented with porn, but the only way I get satisfied is when I stimulate myself anally. I have heard that women sometimes use a candle or banana, would it be safe if I did the same?

You can use whatever you please, as long as it is clean, not too big, has no sharp edges or a rough surface, can't break, or could get lost inside you. With a bit of common sense you can work out what is safe and what's not. To avoid doing any damage put a condom on whatever you choose to stimulate yourself with, apply lots of lubricant, and stop when you feel uncomfortable. But the best thing to do if you want to play it safe and be hygienic is to get an anal stimulator, they are specially designed for the task you have in mind.

I got a couple of geisha balls for an erotic birthday present. They're two silver coloured metal balls, about an inch in diameter. I'm looking forward to trying them out, but what exactly am I supposed to do with them, and what are they good for?

Geisha balls are inserted into the vagina for sexual stimulation. They also train your vaginal muscle and will enhance your ability to exquisitely squeeze and tease your partner's penis with your vagina when you make love.

I am over 50 and have never had intercourse with a woman. At this stage of my life I have given up any hope of finding a woman to be with. I have started to look at alternatives to get some sexual satisfaction. I masturbate a lot, but it doesn't really satisfy me, so I want to try out something new. I have heard about blow up dolls, and found out where I could buy one. I would love to get one, but would that make me a pervert?

No, there is no harm in getting a blow-up doll, and it doesn't make you a pervert. With no woman in your life, it is understandable that you are looking for alternatives to satisfy your sexual needs.

18 Three-some

It seems that Irish people are no longer shy about participating in a ménage à trois – otherwise known as a threesome.

One out of every four Irish people has tried a threesome – sex with another two men or women, at the same time. To make love to and be loved by two partners at the same time is a sexual fantasy that more and more people are playing out.

'I had my first threesome when I was only 18,' confesses Janet (27) from Co. Roscommon. 'I was out one night with my best friend, and we'd met this guy who wanted both of us. At first, I was reluctant, but then I gave in, and had the best night of my life. He had more than enough energy for both of us.'

The classic *ménage à trois* is by no means only enjoyed by swinging singles. Many couples spice up their sex life by inviting a third party into their bedroom. For one out of every 14 Irish couples, threesomes are part of their normal sex life. They share their bed with another man or woman, or go off on their own to enjoy themselves with another couple. The most common form of three-somes is one man with two women, followed by the combination of two men with one woman.

The big question is why can't people be content with one partner? Why do they need two lovers? Some of the many reasons why threesomes are popular are the excitement of something new, people wanting a sexual adventure and the desire to break out of the twosome routine, creating change in a relationship. There is also the kick of voyeurism. The third person in a *ménage à trois* often starts by just watching a couple making love to each other. Then they get involved by touching and kissing the others, and in the end they fully participate in the lovemaking.

The voyeuristic aspect of watching others in the most intimate act of making love, with the prospect of eventually joining in can be a huge turn on. This is one of the main reasons why men especially are so fascinated by the mere idea of threesomes. Some men fantasise about watching two women making love, and then later joining them, to give them the kicks that only a man can offer.

'That was the best experience of my life,' smirks Adam (47) from Co. Galway. 'I brought these two women home from a nightclub. They were best friends, and had played silly sexy games with each other all night to drive me crazy. In bed they started to caress and kiss each other, ignoring me completely. After I had watched them for a while, they took me into their middle, "making a sandwich", as they called it.'

Even though threesomes can be extremely enjoyable and great fun they also have their downsides. Jealousy is often the main problem. Whatever the combi-nation – whether it is two guys with a girl or two girls with one guy, there is always the risk that one of them feels neglected, especially when a threesome isn't a mere one-night-stand, but continues over a longer period of time.

As much as they enjoy threesomes, men find it difficult to share their girl with another guy. Another woman is okay, for she doesn't feel like a real threat. But sharing a woman with another man is something very different – especially when love gets involved.

The same applies to women: sharing a man is fun as long as it is nothing more than sex. But often, after a while, at least one out of the three falls in love – ruining the sexual harmony.

'I have shared my lover with my best friend for a couple of months,' tells Norman (26) from Co. Laois. 'It was great fun for a while, but then the two of them started to get real close, and I was afraid they might both walk out on me. In the end it worked out okay, for my lover decided to stay with me. I would never share her with somebody else again.'

Threesomes can be great fun for a one-night stand or any other kind of sexual adventure – but in the long run, most people prefer the intimacy of the old twosome.

Threesome Types

Now let's look at the best threesome positions, in case you fancy giving a ménage à trois a try!

Two Women and One Man

Two women and one man making love is the most popular way to enjoy a threesome, and there are many ways to make love in this combination. The best variation is two women kissing and fondling each other, then inviting a guy in to share their pleasures. Women often love to play lesbian games to hook their prey. They get the man's attention and then take mercy on him in the end, letting him in on the fun.

Favourite Positions

There are too many two women/one man positions to list them all but here are the most popular ones:

Sandwich *This position is a man's dream. Two women position him in between them. While he makes love to one of them, the other turns towards the couple to share caresses and kisses.*

'I kiss my best friend when we're dancing, like Madonna kissed Britney that night,' explains Valerie (19) from Co. Dublin. 'This never fails to get the guys' attention. Once a guy is hooked, we bring him home and make a sandwich – with him in the middle.'

2 Busy Man *He makes love to one of the women, while he satisfies the other with intimate kisses. Depending on his potency, the women can change roles after the first session.*

3 Triangle *He kisses one of the women intimately, who kisses the other woman, who in turn kisses him. Halfway through the session, everybody has to turn around, so that both women get a taste of his penis, as well as his tongue.*

4 Others *There are many other ways to enjoy a threesome. The women can make love to each other, while he takes one of them from behind. The players can involve vibrators or other sex toys in their encounter.*

'We are two bisexual women who live together,' explains Laura (24) from Co. Dublin. 'Sometimes we feel like sharing a guy for a night. To drive him crazy, we first make love to each other, using a vibrator. Then we let him join in to make love to one of us with his penis, and the other with the vibrator. Of course we take turns, as we both like to come while we feel a real penis inside us. So the guy needs to have a bull's potency.'

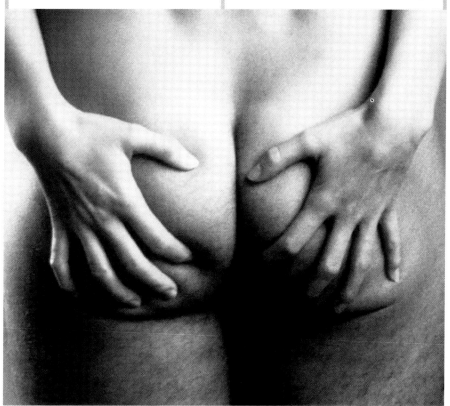

Two Men and One Woman

This is the most satisfying version of a threesome from a woman's point of view. The men sandwich the woman between them and then they take turns making love to her. Or she makes love to both of them simultaneously using her hands and lips.

'My boyfriend doesn't manage to make love more than once per night, and I need more than that, especially as we meet only once or twice per week,' says Carol (32) from Co. Clare. 'So we agreed to let his best friend join us and it worked out great. We kiss and caress each other during foreplay, and then the guys take turns making love to me. Our favourite is me kneeling over one guy, giving him oral sex, while the other one takes me from behind.'

Favourite Positions

1 Sandwich One guy makes love to the woman the normal way, while the other takes her from behind. The easiest technique is to have the first man lie on his back, with her lying or sitting on top of him, and the second guy kneeling between their legs.

If the men are bisexual, one can make love to the woman, while the other guy makes love to him.

Another classic sandwich is when all three lie on their side, both men facing the woman in the middle. This is a very tricky position as it can be difficult for everyone to fit together properly.

2 Give and Take One man has intercourse with the woman, while she manually or orally satisfies the other. This can be especially exciting when they all stand up – she leans over to give the man in front of her oral sex, while the man standing behind her makes love to her.

In another variation, the guy making love to the woman simultaneously satisfies the other man either with his hands or his lips.

'My favourite is to give oral sex to one of the guys, while the other one makes love to me,' describes Astrid (28). 'I meet a couple of lads for this most weekends. They both love to experiment, and we find new ways to make love almost every time we are together. But the best thing about being with two men is that when one gets tired or needs some time to get ready again, there is still another man you can turn to.'

3 Triangle *The woman gives oral sex to one of the guys, who then looks after the other man, while the other man intimately kisses the woman. Again, they need to turn around after a while to make sure everybody gets their fair share.*

4 Others *In the warm up phase to a threesome, both men often kiss and caress the woman, while she takes both of them into her hands. Especially for teenagers, a threesome often starts and ends with mutual masturbation, while older trios normally go for full intercourse. Another pleasurable position is for the woman to have intercourse with one guy, while the other rubs himself between her breasts.*

Three Women

One out of 20 Irish women has tried this out – a threesome with another two women. You can have a sandwich, enjoy oral sex in the triangle position, or two women can rub themselves off each other while they spoil the third one with kisses and caresses. You can use your intuition and imagination to work out the other variations to this threesome.

Sex Dictionary

THREESOME
Sexual act involving three people. Also called ménage à trois.

Three Men

Three guys together can have lots of fun if they are all open-minded, eager and imaginative. Young men often just masturbate each other to find some relief, while more advanced players enjoy a night of unrestricted sex.

A tempting position for this combination is to make love with all three lined up, kneeling behind each other. It is not easy to get in synch in this position, but it can be done.

Most threesomes consist of a couple that has invited a third party in to share the fun.

'My boyfriend and I sometimes invite another guy to stay over with us,' tells Alan (37) from Co. Dublin. 'It gives us new ideas for our partnership. That's how we first got introduced to the pleasures of anal stimulators and penis rings.'

THE THREESOME SURVEY
How many women and men have played threesomes?

	Women	Men
With a woman and a man	8%	9%
With two women	5%	24%
With two men	9%	6%

TIPS

A threesome can be great fun, as long as there isn't any love or jealousy involved.

Don't do anything against your will.

Take precautions so you don't catch STDs.

Q&A

I have had threesomes on a regular basis with a couple of fun-loving girls. Now one of the girls has fallen in love with me, and wants us to be a couple. I like this girl a lot, but I don't love her, and I like the other girl in the same way. What should I do? Is there a chance of keeping both of them? This is what I really want!

Trying to keep both girls would cause you nothing but trouble, so you better end this ménage à trois before the affair turns sour. It might be a small comfort for you to know that most threesomes come to an end due to one or two – or even all three – of the participants falling in love.

My wife wants us to have a threesome with another woman. She confessed that she'd always liked the idea of having sex with a woman. I am afraid of losing her, and nervous that she might be turning lesbian. On the other hand I'm very turned on by the idea. Do I have cause to worry about her sexual orientation?

It is always a dangerous game to invite another person into your marital bed, whether it's a woman or a man. A threesome can spice up your sex life, and therefore have a positive effect on your marriage, but there's also the risk that your partner turns away from you in the end. I'm pretty sure that your wife is suggesting a threesome because she's not fully satisfied in your relationship. So before you indulge in the adventure of a threesome, try to spice up your marital sex life. Spoil your wife in bed. Take your time caressing and kissing her. Ask her what you can do for her. When she says nothing, everything's fine, insist that you'd love to do more. To answer your last question, many women who are in a steady relationship dream of sexual adventures with other guys or girls, but the reason for that is almost always the fact that they feel they're missing out on something in their own relationship.

I would like to try out sex with two men. One of them could be my husband, the other one an eager, adventurous young man. Lately I've being having this fantasy more frequently, but I'm not sure how to present it to my spouse.

The best way to introduce your husband to your idea is to talk about it in a casual way first, to check what he thinks about it, but I'm afraid he won't be enthusiastic about your dream of sharing your marital bed with another guy. Irrespective of your wish to try out a threesome, you should talk to your husband about what's lacking in your relationship from your point of view. He might not even be aware that you aren't sexually satisfied.

The two women I have had an affair with for two weeks have asked me to move in with them. I am very tempted to accept their offer, as sex with them is fabulous. For the first time in my life I got as much sex as I wanted. But I sensed some jealousy between the two of them. This makes me worry that I might get myself into trouble if I decide to live with them.

A threesome can be fun for a one-night stand, a weekend, or a holiday fling, but it's definitely not an ideal situation for a long-term relationship. Jealousy is the main problem, but there's also a good chance that in time you'll prefer one of the women to the other, and wish to be alone with her. This will cause trouble, especially when you live together. Relationships consisting of three people are so unstable and emotionally stressful, that they normally break up after a short while, leaving a broken heart or two behind. As you can sense some jealousy between the two women before you have even moved in with them, you are better off not to accept their offer.

Can two penises be in a woman's vagina at the same time? Is it possible from a technical point of view, and does this happen in threesomes?

It is possible from a technical point of view, although it is a very awkward act that can easily lead to injuries, especially for the female. A more practical and much more common version of a threesome is the simultaneous penetration of the woman's vagina and anus.

I have had a spontaneous threesome with my boyfriend and his best pal. Since that night, I feel strongly attracted to my boyfriend's best friend, and he feels the same way about me. We would like to repeat this experience. The problem is that my boyfriend is strictly against it. He says this threesome should never have happened, and that he has no intention at all of repeating it. What should we do?

Your boyfriend's reaction makes sense, especially as he sees the attraction that has developed between yourself and his pal. He must be afraid of loosing you. You obviously had a great night, and you should leave it at that. Even if your boyfriend agreed to have another threesome, it wouldn't be the same as your first one, as his jealousy would spoil the fun for sure.

My boyfriend and I had a threesome with one of my colleagues. I couldn't believe it: my boyfriend was performing oral sex on him, kissing him all over. Then one night I came

home to find my boyfriend in bed with my colleague, having full-blown sex. He asked me to join in, but I didn't. Sex with him now is wonderful. We try new things all the time. But I can't stop worrying – has my man become gay or bi overnight?

The threesome you have had with your colleague has undoubtedly opened the door for sexual adventures. Your boyfriend is obviously bisexual. He not only was willing to share your bed with another man, but enjoyed having sex with that guy, instead of only watching him making love to you. On the other hand, he enjoys sex with you as well. This fits the classic definition of bisexuality, which is the sexual attraction to persons of both sexes.

Two women, who I thought were lesbians, invited me home for a threesome. I was shy and didn't go with them. But since that night I dream of joining them to see what it's like. Should I go for it if the opportunity comes up again?

Why not go for it if you dream about it? Many men share your fantasy of having a threesome with two women, especially with women who are close to each other, but only a few ever get the opportunity. If you go for it, make sure to give both women the same amount of attention. And don't forget to bring enough condoms.

My boyfriend wants to go to bed with me and my best friend. I know he fancies her, and she is mad about him. I'm afraid they might just do it behind my back if I don't play along and agree to a threesome.

They might fool around behind your back anyway, whether you agree to try out a threesome or not. As you feel that your boyfriend and your best friend are sexually attracted to each other, don't make it too easy for them to get sexually involved. If you agree to share your boyfriend with your best friend, you will basically drive the two of them into each other's arms. In the end you could easily lose both of them.

19 Group Sex

Group sex is still a mystery for most of us. It's certainly not a subject that is talked about in polite society.

We all know that group sex involves several people, more than three, indulging in sexual activities with each other. But who are these folks? Where do they meet? And the big question is what exactly do they do? Let's shed some light on this.

Basically, there are two kinds of group sex enthusiasts. The first type are single men, and to a much lesser extent single women, looking for the opportunity to engage in some sexual activity. The second type are sexually liberal couples looking for sexual distraction from their everyday routine.

Although you don't hear about it often, group sex is far from exotic. One out of every nine Irish men (11%) has tried it, as has one out of every 25 Irish women (4%). One out of 20 couples in Ireland engages in group sex, mainly mature men and women who have been together for a long time. To join in group sex you need to be open-minded, otherwise you spoil the fun for yourself and the rest of the gang.

Group sex parties mostly take place at a member's house. Other meeting places are sex clubs, sex bars and hotels, but private homes are the most favourite places to meet.

'We take turns organising and hosting our parties,' explains Sabrina (45) from Co. Dublin. 'Our group consists of four couples and seven singles who meet regularly. Sometimes somebody brings a guest or two, but mainly we stick to ourselves. I love the private environment. I couldn't relax in a club atmosphere, where most of the people you meet are strangers.'

When a private group sex party starts off, you normally wouldn't know the difference from any ordinary party, like a house warming, a birthday or whatever. There's the usual party atmosphere, with snacks and drinks being served, and people hanging around in small groups having a chat and a laugh. It's only when they start shedding their clothes that things begin to change from the norm and you realise that something different is going on.

Ten is the ideal number of participants. While women prefer a perfect balance between men and women, guys – no big surprise – want women to outnumber the men. Most of the time it is the other way around and there always seem to be a few surplus males on the loose, hoping to pick up some action here and there.

The normal picture of a group sex party isn't ten bodies in a tangled heap, but mainly couples, sometimes threesomes, strewn all over the place, making love, while others stroll around or hang about watching. Many couples strictly stick to themselves, making love with each other in the stimulating atmosphere of the group, allowing others to watch them, while they also observe other couples. While everybody is expected to be tolerant enough to accept and give hugs and kisses, it is not normally expected that everybody is eventually going to end up together.

'My boyfriend and I are best friends with another couple about our age, and on weekends we often stay together and share a bed. While the guys make love to us, we kiss and touch each other. I can't come without my clitoris being caressed, and my best friend has a much better touch than my boyfriend. She never fails to help me come, and I do the same for her.

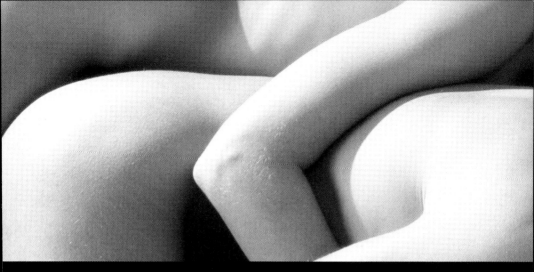

Our guys were startled at first, but by now they have got used to it. They seem to be happy enough that the responsibility of making us come has being taken off their shoulders,' explains Bridie (27) from Co. Longford.

Some group sex parties also involve the 'tangled heap' picture. A foursome with one woman and three guys is very popular at these sessions. This involves a three-way penetration of vagina, anus, and mouth. Another hit is a foursome involving two male/female couples, with the men making love to the women, while the women indulge in pleasing each other.

One out of every six Irish women (17%) and more than every second man (55%) would consider visiting a group sex party, if the conditions were agreeable. The most important condition is a guarantee that nobody suffers from any STDs. The second condition is that nobody is forced to take part in anything they don't want to do. Another major condition for taking part in group sex is that everybody is well-groomed and good-looking.

Nearly one out of five (18%) people in Ireland would be seriously tempted to attend if someone they secretly adore is expected to show up. The assurance of secrecy is also important, many Irish people would attend an orgy but only if they could be sure that nobody else would ever hear about it.

'I went to a group sex party once, because I had heard that the guy I had been after for a good while was going. He had never noticed me before but I thought I might get my chance if I stuck to him and his crowd and joined the party. The nearest I got to him was to watch him having it off with a couple of other women. In the end, I had a good time anyway, as there were more than enough men to console me.' Patricia (31) from Co. Westmeath.

GROUP SEX SURVEY

The answers to the multiple-choice question, 'Under which circumstances would you consider attending a group sex party?' were as follows:

Nobody suffers from STDs	28%
I'm not forced to take part in anything	25%
Everybody is good-looking	19%
Someone I secretly fancy takes part	18%
My attendance stays secret	16%

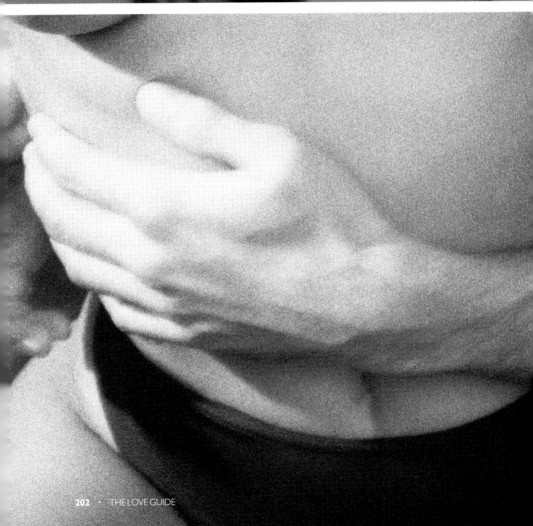

Q&A

My wife and I have decided to spice up our sex life with a bit of group sex. Although I was looking forward to it, I was worried at the same time, and so, I promptly failed to get an erection, which was very embarrassing. I blame this on my strict and demure upbringing. What do you think?

You are probably right. Male sexual potency is mainly controlled by the mind, which allows factors like a prudish upbringing to later influence the adult sex life. But I wouldn't blame your failure to get an erection on your upbringing alone. Group sex is still widely seen as a violation of the existing moral laws of our society. For most of us it is unthinkable to perform sexual acts in the presence of others. This ingrained belief has ruined many planned nights of unrestrained group sex. It you want to go through with your plan, get a prescription for Viagra before you make your next attempt at group sex.

We're a fun-loving little crowd of four couples. Soon we are going on holidays together, and thought that it might be a good opportunity to have a party, and try out some swapping and group sex for a night. Is it safe to do this, or are there any risks involved that we should be aware of?

There are four main risks when it comes to swapping and group sex that you need to be aware of. The first is the possibility of infection with AIDS or other STDs. To avoid any risks to your health, you should always use condoms when you swap partners.

The second factor is the strain group sex might put on your relationships, especially when a 'swapped' couple finds more fun which each other than with their respective partners. If love gets involved, this might even lead to a couple's break up. The third factor you have to take into account is jealousy – one or the other of you might not like the amount of attention their partner gets, or the attention their partner shows to somebody else. Then finally, there is the risk that your fun-loving little crowd will break up over this, as you might feel awkward with each other after your wild night. But enough about the risks – some couples who have tried it say that swapping gave their marital sex life a much needed boost.

My husband and I have been invited to a group sex party. We know the couple who invited us well, and have discussed group sex with them a good few times. We are very tempted to go ahead with it, but don't have a clue about exactly what to expect from such an event.

Talk to the couple who invited you, they definitely know what a group sex party is all about. Meet them for an intimate chat to get informed before you indulge in your adventure.

Does having group sex mean that I have to sleep with everybody who wants me?

No, normally you are free to choose your partners when you have group sex. Of course the other participants expect you to be open-minded and join the crowd, but that doesn't mean that you have to sleep with everybody who wants you. To make sure, check out the rules before you join the group.

Can a single woman participate in group sex or do you need to bring a partner?

A single woman is more than welcome at most group sex sessions. Normally, there is a huge overhang of single male participants, so any single female who wants to join the group will be greeted with cheers.

20 Swinging

When most people think of swinging they imagine a group of couples who share lovers. But swinging is more than the mere sexual involvement of couples with somebody other than their partner. Swingers tend to see their way of living as an alternative lifestyle choice, leaving behind the common moral laws and creating their own.

While most swinging takes place on a couple-to-couple basis, with the full knowledge and mutual consent of all participants involved, single men and women are welcome to take part as well. The aim of swinging is to achieve pleasure and fulfilment, without any emotional attachment getting in the way. Love tends to spoil the fun; so swinging should be based on lust and desire only.

One out of every 25 Irish couples (4%) engages in swinging. Many more are tempted, but either can't muster up the courage, or the right opportunity hasn't arisen yet. One out of every 13 men (8%), and one out of every 14 women (7%) would love to go, but haven't been brave enough yet. For many sexual inhibitions and the strict moral laws they have grown up with are too strong to allow them to consider something like swinging.

'I would love to give swinging a try,' says Audrey (34) from Co. Kilkenny, 'but I wouldn't know where to start. I have checked out the ads in the paper, but they sort of frightened me off, as they were too explicit for my taste. Now I just keep my ears peeled whenever I socialise, and I'm sure the right opportunity will come up one day.'

Swinging Clubs

Most serious swingers are members of a private club that organise events from parties to swinging weekends abroad. While normally membership is required, including a fee, clubs are always on the lookout for fresh blood, encouraging newcomers to join the scene. Single women are usually welcomed with open arms, often without being charged an admission fee. While it's not hard to find willing men to join, it's not easy to recruit a balancing number of women.

Meetings with other swinging clubs are a special treat for every organised swinger, especially attending well-established and experienced clubs in Europe.

'Last summer we visited a small private club in the Netherlands,' tells Moira (37) from Co. Dublin. 'Compared to them, we are real amateurs. It was unreal. The atmosphere was fantastic. In the club garden, everybody ran around naked, completely relaxed. We had a barbecue, a dance, almost like a normal summer's party. The difference being that almost nobody went to bed with their own partner that night. Even during the day, newly found couples vanished into their private rooms, coming back later to join the crowd again, like nothing had happened.'

Not all swinger clubs allow sexual activity on their premises. Some function as a meeting ground only, and leave new couples to find their own bed for the night.

The interest in swinger clubs is immense. One out of three Irish women and four out of ten Irish men does not object at all to swinging clubs. The attitude is a tolerant 'let them swing'. Many people are of course curious about what is going on behind the closed doors of these clubs. Some even make up their minds to check it out but lose their courage at the last moment. The fact that their partner doesn't want to play along is often another one of the main obstacles that keeps open-minded and interested Irish people from swinging.

Rules for New Swingers

If you want to give swinging a try, there are a few simple, but important rules to follow.

1 Seek Your Partner's Consent
The first, and most important rule is that you shouldn't plunge into this adventure unless you have your partner's consent. There is no point in dragging your woman or your man along against their will. It wouldn't be any fun and would almost certainly spell disaster for your relationship.

2 Don't Do Anything Against Your Will
Rule number two is to never do anything against your will. Don't feel under pressure to do something you don't feel up to. If you don't like what is going on, just leave.

3 Be Careful When You Choose A Swinging Club
Check a swinging club out carefully before you commit yourself to anything. You need to keep in mind that some clubs are a facade for hidden prostitution.

4 Don't Get Emotionally Involved
Whenever you are out swinging, try not to get involved emotionally. Swinging is not about love, it is for sexual purposes only.

The Swinging Survey

Irish people were asked the question 'What do you think about swinger clubs?':

	WOMEN	MEN
I'm tolerant – let them swing	33%	41%
I would love to know what's going on there	15%	21%
Would love to go, but can't overcome my inhibitions	7%	8%
My partner refuses to come along	2%	8%
Almost went once, but changed my mind at the last moment	3%	8%

Q&A

A couple my husband and I are good friends with spent a long weekend in a swingers' club in Amsterdam. They told us all about it: how they ran around naked, and how they had unrestrained sex with people they had never met before. When they asked us to come along next time, my husband was all enthusiastic. I am shell-shocked by the mere idea of it. Should I play along to please my husband?

If you find the idea shocking, there is no point in going. Talk to your husband about your reservations. If he is in the mood for experiments, try to think of something exciting you could try out between the two of you instead. If you fulfil another sexual wish for him, I'm sure he won't mind your refusal to try out swinging too much.

My husband wanted to go to a swingers' club. I was very reluctant to go, but in the end I agreed and played along. Although it was my husband's idea to try out swinging, it was me who enjoyed it in the end. He didn't take part in any sexual activity, while I had a great time making love with a young man. Afterwards, my husband started to blame me for enjoying myself, saying that he had watched me, and could tell how much fun I had with the young guy. Not only that, since that night he doesn't sleep with me anymore.

While you had a great time, your husband obviously got nothing but frustration out of your swinging adventure. He was full of plans, but then couldn't get beyond his inhibitions. Watching you having a good time instead of sharing his misery made things worse, so now he takes his frustration out on you. Remind him that you did nothing but go along with his wish, and then just tried to make the best of it once you were there. He has no right to blame you for that. To make it easier for him to recover from his disappointment, assure him that you still love and fancy him.

My husband and I have become good friends with a couple who are into swinging, they often meet other couples to swap partners. So one day they asked us whether we'd be in the mood to try it out with them. I said no thanks, I'd rather stick to my own man, but my husband has been intrigued by the idea. He wants us to give it a try. I have the impression that he fancies this other woman, and wants to do it for that reason only. I would do him the favour and try swinging once, but I'm afraid that I might lose my husband over this. Can you put my mind at ease, or do you think I am right worrying?

The main problem in swinging is the risk of falling in love with the swapped partner, so your concerns are very reasonable. You say that you have the impression that your husband fancies this other woman – do you think she fancies him as well? If yes, you are taking a big risk if you agree to play along.

Can a single woman go swinging, or do you need to bring a partner along?

It depends on the swinger club. Some admit couples only, but most would be more than happy to have a single woman join them.

Do you need to be careful in regard to STDs when you go swinging, or can you be reasonably sure that you are safe?

You have to use condoms when you go swinging. Even if somebody has gone for a check up only recently, he or she could still have AIDS or another infection. Don't trust the others to bring condoms, but bring some yourself.

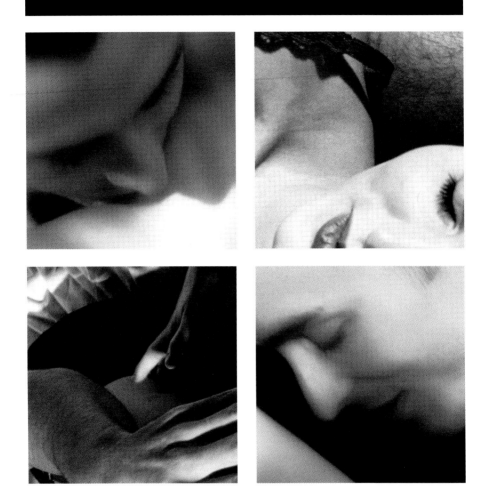

21 Exhibitionism

Exhibitionism has many facets. Initially the term was used to define deviant behaviour in the form of indecent exposure, like exposing your naked genitals to a stranger in an inappropriate setting. Exhibitionism is now also often used to describe love games between couples, which don't cause any harm.

Flashing

The classic picture of an exhibitionist is a guy strolling through the park in a trench coat. When a woman passes by he flashes the coat wide open to expose his naked genitals. The exhibitionist gets a sexual kick out of the look of shock on his surprised prey's face.

Our survey reveals that Ireland has its fair share of exhibitionists. Two per cent of Irish women and three per cent of Irish men admit that they have an exhibitionistic streak and like to expose themselves in front of others. But if you fancy flashing, do it in front of like-minded people. It is unfair and illegal to show off your genitals to a stranger.

'I love to go to the night club wearing only a garter belt under my mini skirt,' admits Deirdre (31) from Kildare. 'When I'm dancing close with somebody, you should see first the shock, then the lust in their eyes when they notice that I'm not wearing any knickers or the gasps when I bend over to pick something up off the floor. My best friend doesn't go out with me anymore since she has found out about this, but I don't mind, I never stay alone long. I always have a small crowd of admirers around me.'

It is much easier for a woman to get away with a little bit of flashing, like this, than it is for a man. A woman can just put her mini skirt on without any knickers in order to do a bit of exhibitionism. It's different for a guy – he has to take more drastic and less innocent measures to flash his bits. Most guys would hardly get a kick out of leaving their fly open and wearing a kilt to play the girl's trick isn't really an option – unless you live in Scotland!

There are many ways, however, for both men and women to live out an exhibitionistic streak within the boundaries of socially acceptable behaviour. You can visit nudist beaches, go to the sauna, join clubs and orgies, or dress provocatively. As long as you don't hurt other people's feelings nobody will mind you flashing.

Games With Your Partner

There is also nothing wrong with living out exhibitionistic fantasies with your partner. You could treat your lover to a striptease. Dress up in a sexy outfit, choose an erotic song you can languidly shed your clothes to, then practice, to get your movements right. As a special treat, wear sexy underwear that shows off your best assets. For an extra kick, you can let your partner take photographs or film you.

'My husband and I are both proud of our bodies, and love to show them off. We take erotic pictures of each other, and sometimes film our lovemaking. When we have the house to ourselves, we play flashing games. My husband for example, would run around with only a towel around his hips, then suddenly let it drop to show off his erect penis. Or he would come home finding me cooking dinner with nothing on but a dress that is so short that half of my bare bum is visible.' Ciara (23), Co Leitrim.

Exhibitionistic games can be great fun, and it is better to live out your exhibitionistic streak with your partner instead of approaching others. It will help to keep you out of legal trouble.

Another way to satisfy exhibition-istic curiosity is to make love in places where other people could discover you. I'm not talking about the shopping centre at lunch hour or a busy beach during daylight. To avoid legal trouble, choose places that are secluded enough to make sure that you don't end up behind bars.

Internet

The Internet is still a relatively new playground for exhibitionists of both sexes. It's not only sex industry professionals who put their intimate pictures onto the net looking for a bit of business. More and more people are posting their pictures online – just for kicks. It's often hard to tell the difference especially if you are new to the game. To play it safe, just stop whenever you are asked for your address, your credit card number or bank details.

'I publish my nude photos on the Internet, showing off my erect penis and all. It is not the same as flashing in front of a live person, but it is fun as well, and at least it keeps me out of trouble. The people visiting my web page don't get there by mistake, they know what they are looking for, and their responses to my pictures keep me going. Some even send pictures back, so my voyeuristic streak gets something out of this as well.' Seamus (47), Co. Cork.

SEX DICTIONARY

EXHIBITIONISM
Getting sexually aroused by exposing oneself in public.

FLASHING
Exposing one's genitals in public.

INDECENT EXPOSURE
Displaying nude parts of the body in a manner that is against local custom and law.

MOONING
Displaying the nude backside, without exposing the front side.

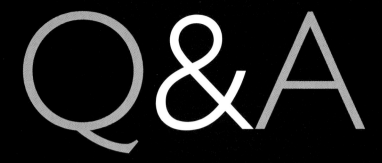

Q&A

I love to show off my naked body. In clothes shops, I undress in the changing cubicle, with the curtain wide open. When guys start gawking at me, I get sexually aroused. The feeling is so intense that I get moist. Does this mean that I'm a pervert?

You obviously have an exhibitionistic streak that means you feel the urge and get aroused by presenting yourself in the nude. Many women love to show off their best assets, and enjoy admiring glances, but your desire goes much farther. If you suffer an urge to undress in public again and again, a psychologist can help to get it under control.

I never wear panties when I go out for a drink. It is hard to explain why I do this; I just love to go nude under my skirt. Only two guys have found out so far, and they found it sexy. My best friend, who found out as well, accused me of being a slut. What is your opinion?

While most men undoubtedly find it sexy when you wear nothing under your skirt, many will agree with your best friend, and say it's sluttish. Even if you don't mean it that way, some will see it as a signal for being sexually available. To avoid misunderstandings of this kind, keep your desire for going bare as private as possible.

I love to send nude pictures of myself to guys I chat to on the Internet. When I told my best friend about this, she said I must be out of my mind to do something so stupid. Our discussion ended in a bad row. Sending my pictures out is great fun, and I don't see how it could be of harm to anybody. What do you think?

Sending out nude pictures won't do harm to anybody, but yourself. And that's the point: if you find it exciting to expose yourself to strangers, you should at least be aware of the possible consequences. You can't know what your chat mates do with your nude photos. The decent guys will keep them for themselves, while others might share them with their friends or worse, post them onto the Internet for everyone to see. If one of your friends or family finds them, word will spread quickly.

I like to let women see and feel my erection. In crowded places I stand close to a woman, then press my erection against her body. When I sit beside a woman on the bus or on a park bench, I touch my genitals through my clothes, or sometimes through the deep pockets of my jeans. If she fails to notice, I start moaning. I can't explain why this game arouses me so much, but I can't stop myself from doing it. It never gets me anywhere with a woman, as they all run away from me as soon as they notice what's going on – some giggling, some embarrassed and others giving me abuse. I'm seriously worried that my habit will get me into trouble one day.

You have to stop harassing women. What you are doing is definitely going too far. It is not only unfair towards the women you approach; it could indeed get you into serious trouble as well. If you can't stop this, you should see a therapist for help.

Is it acceptable to walk around a nudist beach with an erection while you watch others? Or would that be seen as an offence?

You are not supposed to expose a full erection on a nudist beach; too many people would feel offended. If you are lying in the sun and it happens involuntarily, that's not too bad. But you are not supposed to walk around with an erection, gawking at others.

22 Voyeurism

Voyeurism is the act of watching others in the nude, undressing, or performing sexual acts.

The danger of observing covertly, with the added risk of being detected at any time, adds to a voyeur's sexual excitement and pleasure. Voyeurism has as many facets as exhibitionism. The spectrum goes from the absolutely harmless pleasure of watching your partner, to the obsession of having to watch others to gain sexual fulfilment.

Peeping Tom

The classical picture of a voyeur is the 'Peeping Tom' who gazes into people's bedroom windows to catch a glimpse of them in the nude, to watch them undress, or ideally to see them making love. Another version of Peeping Toms are people who cruise lovers' lanes to observe and surprise couples making out in their cars or on nearby grounds. A tourist beach at night is another dreamland for a voyeur, as there is a good chance of stumbling over couples making love, especially if you know the preferred hot spots. You also might encounter the odd voyeur on nudist beaches or any other places where people are naturally naked.

'I have once been to a deserted beach out of season, but it was warm enough to sunbathe in a bikini, which I promptly did. After a while I noticed a guy sitting in the dunes, staring over at me and masturbating.

And I couldn't do anything about it – I was there with my granny of all people – and I didn't want to give her the shock of her life. So I had to pretend I hadn't noticed, but I kept an eye on the guy to make sure that he didn't come any closer. When he was finally gone, my granny started giggling and then said: "I didn't want to say anything as long as he was here, but there was a guy over by the dunes masturbating."'

Peeping Overtly

Another form of voyeurism is the act of watching other people making love with their tacit consent. The extra thrill of working 'undercover' is missing, but instead you get the different kick of being able to watch closely. You can satisfy this type of voyeuristic streak by going to a swingers' club, taking part in orgies, or simply visiting a live sex show.

At sex shows, you see people, mainly men, brimming over with sexual excitement. Nowadays you'll find more and more couples as well, and small groups of open-minded women who are out for a bit of fun and a good laugh.

'My daughter once brought me to a sex show,' tells Rena (56) from Co. Dublin. 'I always wanted to go, but my husband wouldn't even hear of it. So one night out with another woman my age and my daughter, I suggested going to this bar that has live sex. My daughter insisted that she couldn't bring her own mother to a place like that, but in the end she did. We sat there for more than an hour sipping a glass of champagne, first watching a girl dancing around a pole. When we were on our second glass, she was giving oral sex to a guy who later told us he was her husband. Then the guy took her from behind. When he finished, he came over to our table, and asked whether we **would be interested in spending the rest of the night with him. At that stage my daughter dragged us out of there to avoid any further discussions.'**

One out of every 14 Irish people (7%) would love to watch while their partner has sex with somebody else. The preferred method is to invite somebody in for a threesome, and to then watch their partner make love to them. Men above all would love to watch their woman with another woman, while more and more women would love to watch their partner with another guy.

'I find the idea of watching my husband with one of his attractive mates very sexy,' admits Moira (37) from Co. Sligo. 'But he would never agree to that. While he

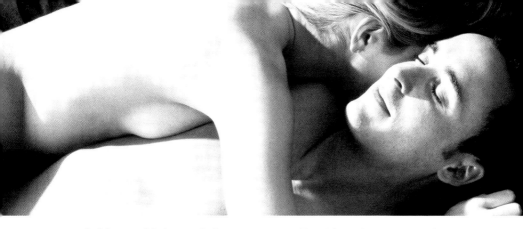

probably wouldn't mind sleeping with another woman and letting me watch. He has once half-heartedly suggested that, but it's out of the question for me.'

Watching Your Partner

The most harmless form of voyeurism is to find pleasure in just watching your partner, or watching the two of you together. Many men dream of watching their women masturbating in front of their eyes, but most women are too shy to play along. It is easier to encourage your partner to striptease or dress up in sexy garments for you. The best way to go about it is to get the sexy underwear yourself, or take her on a shopping spree to make sure the sizes fit, and ask her to try the new outfit on for you later. If you are lucky, you will get a first erotic glimpse in the changing cubicle.

Women also love to see their men in sexy garments instead of baggy briefs with teddy bears or all the other nightmare patterns available.

Buy him what you would like him to wear; most men are very easy going in that regard, as long as they don't feel ridiculous.

Another voyeuristic fantasy many women share is to watch their man ejaculate.

'My wife loves to walk around in the nude while I masturbate, and it really turns her on to see me come. When my wife is not up for sex, she doesn't mind me touching myself. The only condition is that I look at her, and not at some porn. This little agreement is very satisfying for both of us,' reveals Roger (48) from Co. Dublin.

Some women like their partners to masturbate on their belly or their breasts, where they can see everything.

'My boyfriend wouldn't let me watch when he came at first; he was too shy and felt exposed. Now he likes it as much as I do. We sometimes stop making love shortly before he has his orgasm, and I then make him ejaculate over my breasts where I can see him,' says Claudia (25), from Co. Kilkenny.

Watching Your Own Lovemaking

There are many variations in the voyeuristic game of watching your partner and yourself making love. You can choose a position that allows you to watch the most intimate details. Most men's favourite view is to make love from behind, with their women kneeling in front of them. This gives them a very clear picture of what they are doing.

For the female it's much more difficult to watch what's going on. Sitting on top of him with your back towards him, slightly bending over gives you a good glimpse.

Then, you can try out positions in front of a mirror, or better, place two mirrors at a right angle beside and at the top end of your bed.

And last but not least, you can take photographs or film your lovemaking to relive the pleasures later. Using a digital camera guarantees your privacy. Filming you and your partner having sex not only satisfies your voyeuristic fantasies of peeping in on your own lovemaking, it allows you to act out any exhibitionistic streaks you might harbour as well. With the camera's eye zooming in on you, your lovemaking will have another quality.

Sex Dictionary

PEEPING TOM

Another word for 'voyeur', somebody who gets sexually aroused by 'peeping' in on others.

VOYEUR

Somebody who achieves sexual pleasure from watching others, especially from peeping in on people in the nude, undressing or performing sexual acts.

VOYEURISM

Getting aroused by watching or overhearing sexual acts.

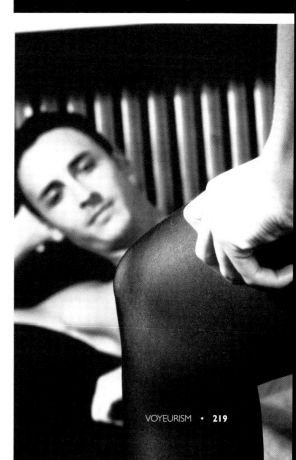

Q&A

My girlfriend caught me watching her having a shower. I have to admit that it turned me on to observe her through the shower doors, as it was a very sexy sight. When she caught me watching, she half-jokingly called me a freaking voyeur. I'm not too sure what exactly a voyeur is, but as far as I know it is kind of a sex pervert. Is that right?

A voyeur is somebody who achieves sexual pleasure from watching others. 'Peeping Tom' is another word for it. A great part of the pleasure is due to observing nudity and sexual activity covertly, with the added risk of being detected.

My boyfriend has a great body, and I love to watch him in the nude. He looks fantastic, but unfortunately he wears absolutely dreadful underwear. How can I tell him how much his baggy boxers turn me off without hurting his feelings? I would really like to see him in something sexy, like a string that shows off his muscular buttocks.

Don't tell your boyfriend how ridiculous he looks in his baggy boxers; just get him the sort of underwear you would like to see on him. Or take him shopping, then point out something sexy, and coax him into trying it on for you. I am sure he'll get the hint without being hurt. It's better not to expect him to wear strings for you all the time; he needs to feel comfortable in his underwear as well. So suggest he wears strings for special occasions.

I want to get some erotic pictures taken of my husband and myself making love. A good friend of mine would take the pictures, but I don't know where to get them developed, I'm worried that our photographs would end up on the Internet. What is the best and safest place to get them developed? I don't mind about the cost, as long as I can be sure that my pictures won't be made public in any way. They are meant for our private pleasure only.

If you don't mind the cost, get a digital camera, and print out your photos yourself. You can get all the equipment you need for less than €1000. That's not cheap, but it's the best you can do to ensure your erotic pictures will stay private. Another option is to use a Polaroid camera, but the pictures won't be of the same quality, and they tend to fade, while digital pictures can be kept practically forever. And you can even digitally enhance their quality.

My hobby is making amateur videos, showing me in bed with former girlfriends and with people I got in contact with over the Internet. My new girlfriend knows about my hobby. The problem is that she finds it abnormal, and refuses to let me film us in bed together. I think there is no harm in doing an erotic video, and later enjoying it together, but she disagrees. How can I convince her that it's okay to play along?

The best chance of you making your girlfriend play along is to grant her full control over the adventure. Let her have the only copy of your sex video, that way she can be sure that it stays completely private. If she still doesn't want to play along, don't put any more pressure on her. I think it is a fair compromise if she lets you keep watching your amateur videos as long as you keep her out of it.

23 Fetishism

Sexual fetishism is not something you hear about very often. When you think about it you often conjure up images of men collecting women's underwear, shoes or more bizarre objects. The meaning of sexual fetishism is the fixation of one's sexual desires on either a part of the body or an inanimate object.

Common fetishes include men and women's underwear; special material like latex or leather; footwear like high heels or boots; body piercing; nappies for grown-ups and many more. Fetishists often get fixated on a particular body part such as breasts, bums, and feet. Most of us feel, at least to some degree, fetishistic arousals, but as long as it doesn't interfere with normal sexual behaviour and satisfaction there is no need to regard it as a problem.

Cross-dressing and Transvestic Fetishism

One of the most common fetishes among men is cross-dressing -- the desire to wear women's clothes, especially their underwear. One out of 25 Irish men (4%) is into it. They wear female clothes to enhance sexual arousal, most of the time without a real partner, but with the fantasy that they play the female part as well. Some cross-dressers long to 'come out' and share their fetish with their partner.

Most cross-dressers are heterosexual males. They collect slips, bras, garter belts, stockings, and other types of lingerie and night-clothes. Many men love the feeling of silk or nylon on their skin, so they wear these garments to fulfil their fantasy. Some also like to look at themselves in a mirror when they are dressed up; others even take photographs to relive the scene later on.

Some men go no further with their cross-dressing than wearing women's lingerie under their external male clothing. For them it is a way of getting a bit of comfort in a stressful world.

Many experts agree on the fact that cross-dressing comes within the normal range of male sexuality, as long as it doesn't become an obsession that takes over your life. Lots of people cross-dress occasionally – women and men alike. For women it is easy enough to get away with it. A woman can wear boxer shorts, or even put on a suit and tie without anybody getting upset. For men it is a different story, and, as much as I hate to say so, not completely without reason.

A woman who slips into her guy's boxers and shirt simply thinks it makes her look cute, but in most cases there is no sexual excitement involved, other than maybe feeling a bit closer to her guy. But, a guy putting on his girlfriend's underwear is well aware of the fact that he only looks cute to himself and other like-minded fellows. Maybe he would love to share his desire with his girlfriend, but he knows very well that revealing his fetish would most likely end in trouble.

And then, a man's desire normally doesn't stop with just wearing his lover's panties. The main idea is to use them for masturbation. Again, there is nothing wrong with that, but another injustice between the sexes strikes at this point. When a man masturbates he leaves sticky and unmistakable evidence behind, while a woman can satisfy herself without leaving a trace.

Why Do People Cross-dress?

People cross-dress for a wide variety of reasons. Some do it just for fun, others want to make a point against the established rules of morality and etiquette in society, while most do it just to live out their own fantasies and desires.

The main problem is that girlfriends and wives find it hard to understand why their men would want to dress up in female gear. So the main problem for a cross-dresser is how to get his partner to play along, or how to at least make her accept his fetish.

Telling Your Partner

The best way to bring the issue up is to have a playful go at it. Buy your lover a couple of sexy outfits and then ask her to try them on. Playfully try one on yourself and see how your lover reacts. If she plays along that's great, and if she doesn't you can still back off, pretending that you tried her garments on only for fun.

Introducing cross-dressing into a relationship can allow the relationship to become more intense and intimate, or it can put it at severe risk, eventually causing it to fall apart. It is not advisable to confront a new partner with your fetish at the beginning of your relationship, but you should do it before your relationship becomes really serious. If your partner can't accept your fetish, it is easier to break up early, than having to go through the break-up of a long-term relationship or even a marriage. Being rejected, at an early stage, doesn't hurt as badly as it would once the relationship has matured and you have developed a strong bond with your partner.

Unfortunately, the rate of rejection is high, as the majority of women don't fancy making love to a guy who is dressed up in women's clothes. They are put off by the idea, or even find it alarming. But then, the odd woman doesn't mind, or even sees it as a turn on.

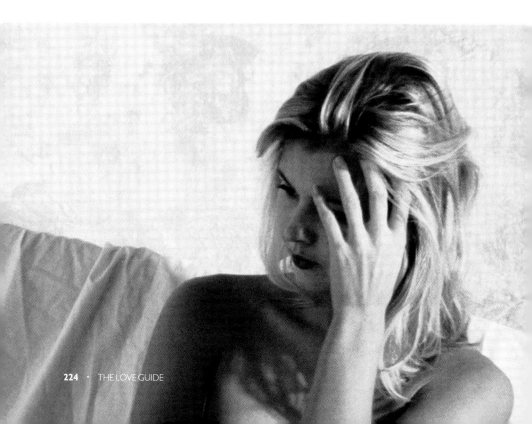

A Few Fetishes

Foot Fetishism *A foot fetishist finds sexual excitement and fulfilment by watching, touching, or kissing somebody's feet. Some also like being masturbated by their partner's feet.*

A foot fetishist reacts to feet like another person would to the sight and handling of genitals. While some prefer bare feet, others add a shoe fetish, stocking fetish, or different variation to their general sexual attraction to feet. Some prefer high heels, others love stockings or find leather boots or any other type of footwear a big turn on. It is often difficult to distinguish between foot fetishism, shoe fetishism, stocking fetishism and others, as they are often combined.

'My husband is a foot fetishist,' explains Elizabeth (33) from Co. Dublin. 'His favourite thing to do is to caress my bare feet. He gives me long massages and pedicures. He loves to paint my toenails and then he makes me wear high heels when we make love. I have to circle his bum with my legs and press my heels into his buttocks, so firmly, that it hurts.'

Rubber Fetishism *A rubber fetishist is sexually attracted to rubber garments. This is closely related to latex and PVC fetishism. These shiny materials form a second skin, which seems to be part of the kick. To wear a tight rubber outfit gives you the feeling of being caught in a second skin. The sensation of being peeled out of it is especially intimate, as you are literally shedding your skin, completely exposing yourself. The person wearing rubber or similar garments is as good as naked; all their body's contours are clearly visible – another big turn on for many people. While a majority of rubber fetishists fancy extremely tight and skin-like garments, others like wide cloaks, preferably transparent ones.*

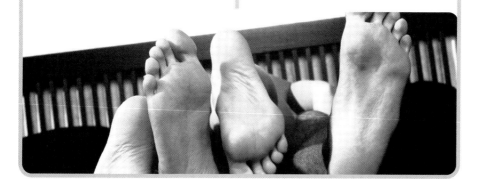

'My husband loves to wear a transparent suit bag, the ones you sometimes get from the dry cleaners,' admits Laura (48) from Co. Longford. 'He has found one that is big enough to fit both of us in, and we sometimes wear it when we make love. I first found it a bit stupid giving in to his wish, but I got used to it, and don't mind anymore, as long as it makes him happy.'

Rubber fetishists can be attracted to other garments including everything from Wellingtons to raincoats, divers' suits to shower curtains. It is a wide field that provides the fetishist with lots of new pleasures, especially if they are into experimenting.

There's a very substantial and specialised industry that serves the rubber fetishists' needs, producing specialised clothing and articles. You also find magazines that specialise in rubber fetishism. There are an amazing amount of support groups for people who have problems in dealing with their fetish, or think that it is getting out of hand.

3 Nappy Fetishism

Nappy fetishism is a form of infantilism where the player, almost always a male, gets sexually stimulated and finds relief in wearing nappies. Some men play on their own, wearing the nappy until it becomes necessary to change it, then masturbating over a fantasy that some nanny or nurse comes and cleans up their mess.

There are many variations to this game. Some lucky ones have a partner who plays along, scolding them while they tidy them up as part of their role playing, while most have to look after themselves in the end.

4 Other

Other quite common fetishes include medical fetishism, tickling fetishism, and leather fetishism. The name basically gives away what it is all about. It is a bit trickier when it comes to depilation fetishism – that means to get sexually excited by removing body hair.

Less common are milk fetishism – the kick of drinking human milk – and eyeglass fetishism. Hard to believe, but not everybody wearing glasses really needs them. Some people out there wear glasses for sexual stimulation.

'The strangest thing I have ever come across was a guy who had perfect eyesight, but used to borrow glasses from other people in public for just a second or two, explaining that he forgot his own glasses at home, and can see next to nothing without them. So he would borrow glasses from a guy at the bookies to fill out his betting slip, or from an old lady at the bus stop to check out the timetable. And what's even stranger is that it turned him on,' says Fiona (27) from Co. Dublin.

Sex Dictionary

CROSS-DRESSING
Wearing clothing of the opposite sex for sexual stimulation and satisfaction.

DEPILATION FETISHISM
Getting sexually aroused by the removal of body hair, for example shaving or waxing.

FETISHISM
Sexual fantasies, urges, and behaviour that involve objects like undergarments or boots, or special body parts, like a person's feet to enhance sexual arousal.

FOOT FETISHISM
Showing sexual interest in human feet.

MEDICAL FETISHISM
Sexual fascination with medical activities and objects, like intimate examinations and procedures such as prostate massage.

RUBBER FETISHISM
Getting sexually aroused by wearing garments made from rubber, or watching or touching others wearing them.

TICKLING FETISH
Getting sexually aroused from being tickled, or by tickling a sex partner. Often used in combination with restraints.

WATERSPORTS
Sexual fascination with urine, like peeing in public, being peed on or peeing on others.

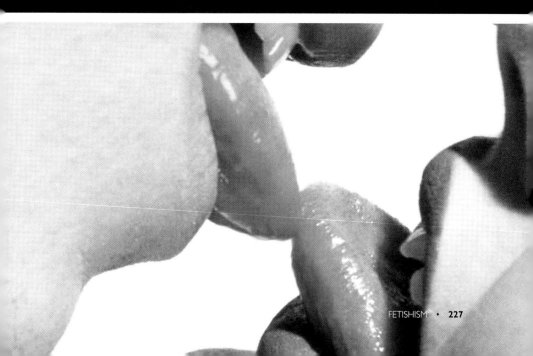

Q&A

A lady I have been seeing lately had an awful go at me when she found out that I secretly wear stockings and a garter belt. The scene couldn't have been any worse – she caught me masturbating in front of the bedroom mirror. She accused me of being a fetishist, and said that she doesn't want to see me ever again. I am hurt that she accuses me of being a pervert, isn't it harmless what I'm doing? I am only having a bit of fun with myself. I don't molest anybody!

A fetishist isn't a pervert, it is a person who has an erotic fixation on a special part of the body or an object, like clothing or footwear. I agree that what you are doing is harmless, but you have to try to understand your lady friend as well. It must have been quite a shock for her to see you masturbating, dressed up in a garter belt. Give her some time to overcome her shock, then try to talk to her about your feelings. She might be understanding.

Since the age of 17, I have had the habit of nicking my mother's panties and masturbating over them. My mum found out about this years ago, but after yelling at me once, she has never brought the subject up again. Now I go much further, I secretly wear my mum's lingerie, even during the day. I feel bad for fancying my own mother's lingerie in a sexual way, but there's nothing I can do about it. What is wrong with me?

You are too fixated on your mum, but I'd say that your main infatuation is with female lingerie, and your mum's stuff is conveniently at hand. A guy should go out and meet girls his own age instead of projecting his sexual needs and desires onto his beloved woman at hand – his mum. I think it's time that you cut yourself loose from your too close relationship. To become more independent, it would be a good move to find a place of your own to live in.

You might not think that this is a serious sex problem, but it concerns me very much, so I hope you can help me. My boyfriend spent his college years in Arizona, USA and brought back a pair of genuine, handmade leather cowboy boots to remember his years over there. The problem is that he loves to wear them in bed. I'm not fussy, but this is a bit too macho for my taste. What do you think? And what should I do about it?

It is a bit macho, all right. There are two things you can do about it. First, tell him how much it turns you off, and ask him to come to bed barefoot. As a special kick, let him wear those boots from time to time, but not on a regular basis. The other option is to get a pair of boots yourself, and wear them in bed to make him understand your point of view. But be prepared – he might love your boots, and then you'll be even worse off.

I robbed a pair of knickers from a woman I fancy. This isn't the first time that it has happened; I've done this with other women as well. Normally I get the knickers, go to the toilet, and masturbate. But this time I didn't have enough time, so I kept her knickers. What should I do about this?

There is nothing wrong with getting a thrill from women's knickers, but you shouldn't make a habit of robbing them, as tempting as it might be. Although your little fetish is harmless, most women would be pretty upset if they found out what you are up to with their underwear. So I'm torn between scolding and reassuring you – scolding for invading these women's privacy, and reassuring you that it's pretty normal, only that most men wouldn't have the courage to own up to it.

Except from a few brief encounters with prostitutes abroad, I have never had sex, although I am over 40. One of the ladies once put me in nappies. It was so exciting that I want to wear nappies all the time now. Do other men feel the same? And what should I do when I meet a woman I like? I'm afraid she won't understand my strange desire.

You are not the only one who fancies wearing nappies, but unfortunately, it's almost exclusively men who indulge in this sexual fantasy and play. So you are right, most women would be strongly put off by a guy who wears nappies for sexual pleasure. It's very unlikely that you'll find a woman who shares or even accepts your fetish. So don't reveal your fetish to a new partner, but try to enjoy more widely accepted sexual pleasures to avoid disappointment and frustration. Later on you can still playfully try to introduce them to your fetish.

My husband is a bit odd to say the least. I found out a few years ago that he loves to wear women's clothes. He dresses up in bras and panties, and sometimes masturbates wearing my lingerie; strangely this always gets him into the mood to sleep with me. More and more, he pretends to be a woman on a lesbian fling on those occasions, and this makes me worried. Maybe he's gay, and all this play-acting means that he really wants to be with another man?

I get many letters from married men who love to dress up in female underwear, especially bras, panties and stockings. Most of them want to be with their wife when they do it, although they play a female role themselves. These men aren't gay, but simply out for some kinky games with their lover. As long as it doesn't become an obsession, I see cross-dressing as a harmless fetish that can enhance people's sex lives.

For a couple of years now I have suspected my husband of secretly wearing my lacy thongs. Yesterday I found some shocking proof, semen traces in a thong that I definitely haven't worn yet. My first reaction was utter disgust and shock; I wanted to leave my husband on the spot. But then I began to have second thoughts, leaving me confused and not knowing what to do. I haven't confronted my husband yet about his perverse actions, not knowing how to bring it up. Our marriage has always been happy, and I don't want it to end like this.

Don't end your marriage over this. Your husband obviously has secretly been using your thongs for a good while, without negative effects on your marriage. If you are happy together, try to accept your husband's fetish. It might be best not even to talk about it. But if you feel like confronting your husband, try not to blame him, but be matter-of-fact to avoid an emotional conflict. To clear the air, an open talk is much more helpful.

My husband always wears my aprons when he is doing housework. I wanted to get him a man's apron, but he said he'd rather have mine. I have never seen a man wearing a woman's apron. I think it looks very odd.

I guess you're wondering whether your man is cross-dressing? He might actually like to slip into a female role now and then, but it's much more likely that he just doesn't care whether he's wearing a woman's or a man's apron. Anyway, don't spoil your husband's fun, let him wear your aprons if he likes. It might look a bit odd, but it is completely harmless.

I am absolutely mad about long, black leather boots. My former girlfriend used to wear them to turn me on, and the sex we had when she was dressed up like that was fabulous. Now that she's left me, I cut pictures of girls wearing long black boots out of magazines. Sometimes I hang out in shoe shops. I've even asked a girl to try boots on for me, pretending I was looking for a birthday present for my girlfriend. Would you say I'm a fetishist?

I would worry about fetishism only if something like loving boots becomes an obsession, this means if you're seriously overdoing it. I can't see any harm in your fancy for long boots, but you shouldn't ask girls to try them on for you, as they'd feel awful if they caught you leering at them.

For the past 20 years I have been on my own, and had to masturbate to find sexual release. I got into the habit of wearing female clothes and underwear to turn me on but now I have met a wonderful woman at last and although I really fancy her, I can't come when we sleep together. I secretly dress up in women's underwear when she has fallen asleep, and then touch myself. Should I tell my lady friend?

It's better not to tell your lady friend that you can only come when you wear women's underwear, as there is a great risk that it would frighten her off. Having been alone for almost 20 years, you are fixated on your usual method of sexual satisfaction. It will take some time, but now that you have a lady friend, you will eventually learn to find satisfaction with her. For a start, why don't you get her some sexy lingerie to dress up in?

All my friends fancy guys who don't have much body hair, while I myself like my men hairy. I love to play with the body hair, and enjoy feeling its touch against my skin. My friends always slag me, saying I'm not normal. What do you think? I have to say that I'm quite hairy myself.

Body hair is one of the indicators of masculinity, so it is natural for you as a female to feel attracted to it. But like many other basic instincts, fancying hairy guys is not fashionable. Right now, androgynous, part masculine/part feminine looking guys are in vogue, while 30 years ago men were wearing breast hairpieces to impress women. So the best you can do is to stick to your own instincts and feelings, don't let them being dictated by fashion.

My girlfriend has long brown hair. I always love it when she lets it down, but now I have seen her hair wet, and that looked so sexy that I more or less dragged her out of the shower to make love to her. She was amused by my sudden love attack, but afterwards asked what came over me. I cannot explain it. Should I be worried about this? Or do other guys feel the same?

A naked, wet woman in the shower is a classic erotic scene, so it's no wonder that you fell for it. That the strong erotic signal didn't come from your girlfriend's naked body, but her wet hair, is not so unusual. We all have our favourites – some like long legs, big breasts, tiny waists, or full hips – and you fancy long wet hair. I can't see anything wrong with that, and it's definitely not strange or even perverse.

For the past two years I have been buying sexy underwear for my wife, so I could wear it myself on the sly. It worked fine until only a few days ago, when she caught me wearing her bra and garter belt. To make things worse

I was playing with myself when she saw me. My wife made a big scene, accusing me of being a pervert, and not loving her anymore. She has hardly talked to me since, and avoids me whenever she can. What can I do to save my marriage? Would it help to promise her never to wear her lingerie again?

You need to talk openly to your wife. Try to explain that your fondness for female underwear is a harmless fetish that has nothing to do with your feelings for her. I hope she will accept it, and let you have your fun. If she doesn't, don't make any promises that you can't keep. Better say that you will try to give your fetish up, and just be even more discreet about it if you can't stick to it.

When I first slept with my new man, I was surprised at how smooth his legs were. There is no hair on them at all. The same goes for his chest and armpits. I teased him about it, and he admitted that he shaves his legs, his chest and armpits. Not only that, he confessed that he loves to wear silk underwear and nylons. This has me deeply troubled. I love this man, but at the same time I'm afraid that he is a weirdo.

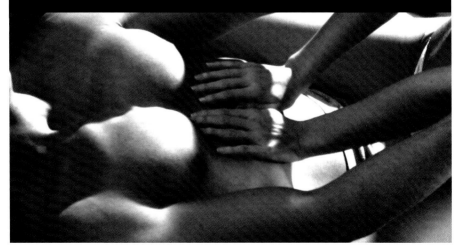

Men who shave and cross-dress are not as unusual as you might think. Many guys fancy it, but are afraid to do it. Others secretly wear women's clothes behind their lover's backs because of the fear of being found out. Most of them long to be honest. Your man at least didn't deceive you in any way; he has been open and true about his fetish. So be open minded, talk to him about his desires and your concerns. If you love each other, and you can manage to tolerate his fetish, I can't see why it should keep you from building a loving and caring relationship.

I am mad about women's feet. When I see a woman, I first glance at her feet and ankles, while other men probably look at a woman's face or breasts first. I love to kiss my girlfriend's feet, but she never lets me do it, although she admits that she likes it herself. She says it's humiliating for me, but I think that is stupid. What is your opinion?

I can't see why you shouldn't kiss your girlfriend's feet. It is not humiliating to do something that you both enjoy. Sure, it is an unusual desire, but you should both feel lucky to be able to share it with each other.

When I sneaked into my boyfriend's apartment to give him a nice surprise, I got the shock of my life instead. He was sitting in front of the telly, wearing nothing but a T-shirt and a nappy while watching hardcore porn. We know each other for more than a year, and I didn't have a clue that anything was wrong. I split up with him, but now I'm having second thoughts. I think I might have been too impulsive. I love him very much, and would stay with him if I could be sure that something like this would never happen again.

There is no guarantee that it will never happen again. I can understand that you were shocked at seeing your boyfriend enjoying himself wearing nappies, but he is entitled to some understanding as well, even if this sexual preference seems to be a bit unusual. If you want to stay with your boyfriend, you need to be tolerant towards his ways, and at least talk to him about it. And don't forget that you walked in on him when he believed that he had a few private moments to himself.

I find a woman's feet one of the most erogenous parts of her body. I get sexually aroused when I see a slender foot in high heel sandals, or a bare pedicured foot. At home I have a huge collection of second-hand pumps and sandals. My last long-term girlfriend didn't have a problem with it. She even brought me to an orgasm with her feet. Since we split up four years ago, I haven't had much luck with women. I'm afraid my peculiar desire is to blame for that. I admit to being a foot fetishist, but is that so bad that I have to stay on my own? The last woman I brought home even called me a pervert before she stormed out of my apartment. Why can't women be more tolerant?

There is nothing wrong with being mad about women's feet, and there are actually many guys who share your feelings. The problem is that your desire is so intense and obvious, that women are taken aback. This is by no means a sign of female intolerance. I'm sure that most men would feel a bit uneasy as well about a woman who displays a huge collection of worn men's shoes at home. To improve your chances with women, try not to be too fixated on your fetish. Give a woman a chance to know you better before she learns about your sexual preferences.

My husband always loved to suckle my breasts. Now that I have had a baby he is at my breasts all the time, not only nibbling my nipples but also taking sips of my milk. I can tell by his erection that it turns him on big time, and I enjoy it as well, although my breasts are a bit too sensitive at the moment. Is there any harm in what we are doing? And do you know whether other couples do the same?

There is no harm in what you are doing, so if you like it yourself, let your husband suckle your breasts if it turns him on so much. You're not the only couple who enjoy this love game. Often men lust after their women's breasts even more when they swell with pregnancy and childbirth. Women have mixed feelings about this. Some feel too sensitive and sore to play along; others are reluctant to give in to erotic longings, being too focused on their babies. But more and more young mothers feel like you do, and simply enjoy their special erotic feelings.

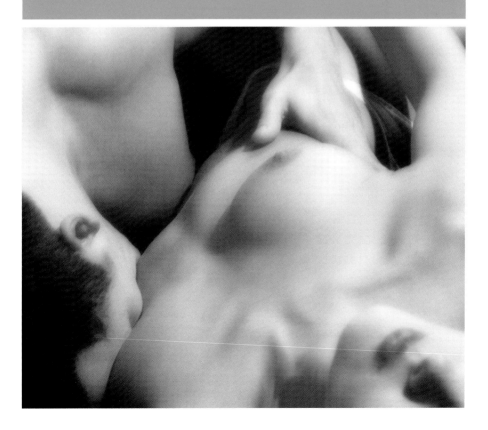

24 Playing Rough – BDSM

You can find all subgroups and major techniques of BDSM in the acronym itself.

B&D – Bondage and Discipline

B&D play is the combination of Bondage and Discipline. The bondage part can be anything from a harmless tying to the bedposts with a soft scarf, up to chains and locks that leave you helpless. Discipline can be anything from having to provide some sexual or non-sexual service to your partner, to being whipped or otherwise punished.

D&S – Dominance and Submission

The person playing the dominant role takes charge of the play, while the submissive part obeys. This play can be extended to outside the bedroom, in the form of a master and slave role play to get into the mood for the final scene.

S&M – Sadism and Masochism

Sadomasochistic play includes B&D and D&S, as well as English play, sex games involving violence or flagel-lantism. The wide range of garments and utensils used include leather gear, shackles and whips. Inflicting and bearing pain is part of the game.

The sadist is the one who finds sexual pleasure from inflicting pain and dominating others, while the masochist enjoys the same on the receiving end.

What is it all about?

The practices involved in BDSM are about inflicting and suffering physical restraint, humiliation and pain. All this is done with the mutual consent of all participants, aiming not at sexual abuse, but at mutual pleasure and fulfilment. Play it safe. Always agree on a safety word when you play BDSM. Take turns playing the dominant and the submissive part to ensure that your sex play doesn't affect the balance of power in your relationship.

While there is a steadily growing community who regard BDSM play as much more than special

techniques to find sexual fulfilment, but as a different lifestyle of their own, most people who enjoy a bit of bondage, pinching, or playing rough do it for mere pleasure without any other implications.

Safety

For whatever reasons you enjoy BDSM – it is important to stick to the rules of safety and mutual, informed consent. Talk about what you are about to act out, clarify the exact rules and how far you are willing to go. Always agree on a safety word that immediately stops whatever activity is going on. This will make sure that you get out of situations that go too far or even become seriously dangerous.

Outside the BDSM community, the factor of discipline doesn't have much impact in rough play. It is mainly bondage that couples enjoy. Bondage is one of the sex practices that has become quite popular. One out of every seven couples (14%) love to tie each other up for sex. They use everything from scarves, ties and robes, to handcuffs and chains, to tie themselves to bedposts or to perform even fancier restrictions.

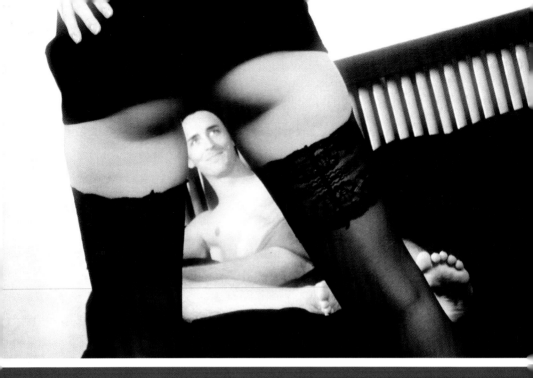

Sadomasochistic sex games are also growing in popularity. These games involve the infliction of pain or at least the threat of it. This does not include severe beatings or torture. It is only a very small minority that's up to that. Most stick to playful biting, scratching, slapping, and rough sex in general. 43% of women and 52% of men have had lustful experiences with pain, mainly with gentle slaps or rough intercourse, but some heavier stuff as well.

Bondage

While members of the BDSM community see bondage as a technique of power exchange, for the 'rest' of us bondage is just one of the games that spice up our sex life.

The most popular form of bondage is tying your partner's wrists to the bedposts with a soft scarf or tie. More adventurous couples use anything from a rope up to handcuffs, or even chains. In a rare variation of this game, the ankles are tied to the bedposts as well, leaving the 'victim' spread-eagled and vulnerable, depending on the partner's mercy. Most couples wisely use means of bondage that the victim can escape from without too much trouble, or otherwise agree on a safety word to stop the game in case it goes too far.

There are uncountable ways and techniques of tying up your partner for the game. An experienced BDSM player probably knows more knots.

than a sailor. But for beginners and players who don't take it too seriously, a simple scarf or a tie around the wrists will do for starters. To increase the intensity of the play, the submissive partner can be blindfolded, or the dominant partner can wear a mask to pretend anonymity.

The main point of bondage is the playful submission of a partner, to play-act the role of a sex slave. As long as it doesn't get out of hand, and that basically means, as long as the submissive part of the bondage game can get out of it any time they want to, there is nothing wrong with it. Most people find if it's kept playful, bondage is fun. But only try it with a partner you absolutely trust, otherwise it can turn into a nightmare.

'I would never engage in bondage with anybody but my husband,' says Sylvia (39). 'I know he would never overstep the rules we have agreed on. I trust him so much that I even let him put me into a straightjacket the other night. It was fantastic; almost a bit too much dependency to bear, but my Tom didn't let me down. And anyway next time, it's him wearing the jacket...'

Inflicting Pain

Pain acts as a sexual stimulant for many of us, as long as it is dished out in small quantities, not really hurting, but only bordering on the threshold of real pain. Sure, there's a few who go over the limit and find pleasure from inflicting or receiving severe pain, but that is the exception rather than the rule since S&M now has become a less extreme, and more fun oriented sex game.

Nibbling and Biting

On average, two out of every five women and every second man have had lustful sexual experiences involving pain. The favourite is nibbling and biting – 31% of women and 24% of men classify love bites as lustful. They can make you shiver with the most exquisite pleasure, provided your lover keeps his teeth in check, and doesn't tear chunks out of you. A nibble on the neck or shoulder, turning more urgent with the progress of your love play, can be a real turn on – just make sure to stop when your partner starts showing signs of distress.

Slapping

The survey results revealed that gentle slaps are the second most lustful experience with pain in Ireland.

'I absolutely love it when my wife slaps my naked bum', confesses Derek (43). 'It's like she is urging me on when I make love to her, especially when she uses the small whip we got her from a sex shop.'

Scratching

One out of every five people loves scratching. The secret is to get the pressure right. You need to put your nails deep enough into the skin to make it hurt a bit, at the same time making sure that you don't draw blood, as that would definitely spoil the fun. The best zone to scratch is the back and bum, and if you can keep it gentle enough, the inner thighs.

Squeezing and Pinching

Be very gentle with squeezing and pinching your partner's genitals, even when you are into rough play. More women than men like this sort of stimulation, for the simple reason that rough caresses can be extremely painful if they involve a man's genitals, to be more specific, a man's testicles. The penis can take a firm squeeze, but the testicles need to be treated with a lot of caution, as a hearty squeeze can bring tears of severe pain even to the toughest guy's eyes, ruining even the best game.

Rough Intercourse

One out of every four women, and more than two out of every five men fancy rough intercourse. That means to just take the partner, or being taken, going for animalistic instincts rather than sensual love play. Rough sex more likely than not leaves you sore and bruised, but now and then it is a great way to release all your sexual tension.

'I wish my husband would go for it more often,' complains Nina (22). 'But he thinks it is his duty to always spoil me with a long foreplay, and then make love to me tenderly. And all right, normally that is the way I like it, but now and then I wish he would just take me whatever way he fancies. Last time I coaxed him around to go for it, he was full of apologies next morning when he saw a couple of bruises on my inner thighs. But I felt great, and didn't mind them at all.'

The Results

Did you ever have lustful sexual experiences involving pain?

	WOMEN	MEN
Yes	43%	52%
No, pain has never turned me on	31%	28%
Never tried it	26%	20%

Which of the following love games do you find arousing?

	WOMEN	MEN
Scratching	22%	18%
Nibbling and biting	31%	24%
Gentle slaps	20%	25%
Rough intercourse	26%	43%
Rough grabbing	13%	12%
Hard squeezing or pinching of genitals	10%	7%
Dominance	23%	12%

Sex Dictionary

BONDAGE
Practice or act to restrain freedom of movement.

CLAMPING
Pinching sensitive areas like nipples or genitals with clamps. There are a variety of specially designed clamps for that purpose.

COLLAR
Worn around the throat, often designed to attach a leash.

FLAGELLATION
Another word for whipping.

SAFE WORD
A word or action given by the submissive to stop the activity.

S&M
Abbreviation for sadism and masochism, meaning to find sexual pleasure by inflicting pain (sadism) or enduring it (masochism).

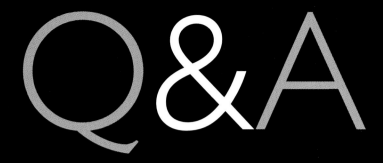

Q&A

It gives me immense pleasure when my wife dominates me in our love life. She didn't want to play along at first, but then we started playing bondage, with her tying my hands to the bedposts. We got her a black corset and long black leather boots to dress up in for our games. Sometimes she uses a small whip on my bare behind to playfully punish me for disobedience. So far so good. But now she has bought a collar and leash, and that is going too far for my taste. I would feel stupid being led by her on a leash. On the other hand, I don't want to disappoint her, as she always tries to fulfil my wishes.

Are you sure it is your wife's true wish to put you on a leash? She might have bought those utensils not for her own pleasure, but mainly to please you, knowing how much you love being dominated. Why don't you have a word with your wife to check this out? If she really fancies putting you on a leash, it might be a good idea to consider it before you dismiss the idea altogether. After all, it can't be much worse than being whipped on your bare behind.

My girlfriend, who is much more sexually experienced than I, wants us to try bondage, but I'm not sure what exactly she means by that. So I checked on the Internet, and found a broad spectrum of sadomasochistic practices there that come close to torture, involving whips, chains and the infliction of pain. I find it hard to imagine that my girlfriend could fancy anything like that.

It looks like you got the wrong picture. The practices you describe sound like strict B&D – Bondage and Discipline, where one person is physically restrained, while another applies all sorts of 'disciplining' and humiliating abuse. I am sure that your girlfriend has something completely different in mind. There is a playful and much more popular version of bondage, where a partner is bound not to inflict pain or humiliation, but just to enhance sexual excitement by play acting.

It started with an affectionate slap on her bum when my wife rode me in bed. It turned her on so much that she now wants me to hit her harder, which of course I've refused to do. The other day she brought home a small whip and asked me to whip her bum while she straddles me. I was shocked, and angrily refused to use the whip on her. Did I do the right thing? Or should I play along, even if it repels me?

You were right not to fulfil your wife's masochistic fantasy. Castigation is a dangerous game. Although your wife might beg for it one moment, she might feel mistreated and mortified the next. If you don't want to let her down completely, give your wife harmless, light slaps on the bum. That way, she can fantasise about being beaten, while you can be reassured that you don't really hurt her.

I achieve the most intense orgasm when I can scratch and bite a man while we make love. Already two boyfriends have left me because of it. But I just can't help myself. When I get aroused I start scratching my lover's back and bum and biting his neck and shoulders. What can I do?

While most men aren't crazy about being scratched and bitten while they have sex, some men love it, at least as long as you don't draw blood. If this slightly sadistic sex game gives you so much pleasure you shouldn't give up. Although you have experienced two failures already there is a good chance that you will eventually find a man who shares your sexual preferences.

My new boyfriend is very voracious in his lovemaking, and I'm afraid that he might have an abnormal streak. Every time we sleep together, he starts to nibble on my shoulder or neck shortly before he reaches his orgasm. When he comes, he sinks his teeth into my flesh while he groans deeply. These bites don't really hurt, and they rarely leave a mark on me. I have to admit that I enjoy them, although I find my boyfriend's behaviour deeply disturbing at the same time.

Don't worry, there is nothing wrong with your boyfriend or yourself. Love bites are a normal part of a passionate sex life.

When I kiss my partner all over I like to nibble on his naked flesh and gently bite him. He loves the kissing part, but he hates it when I use my teeth, saying the pain spoils it for him. Especially when I get near his privates I can feel him go all tense instead of relaxed. I think he is being a sissy, but he says that any kind of nibbling in that area is very painful. Could that be true, or is he exaggerating to stop me doing this?

Nibbling and biting in that area can indeed be painful, especially when you go near his testicles. Your poor man can't relax when you attack him like that. As soon as you get near his most tender spots, he naturally gets tense, expecting to feel your teeth any moment. If you love nibbling so much, let your boyfriend show you where it's okay to nibble, and where it causes him discomfort.

I love to slap my husband's bum when we make love. It is like firing him on to take me harder. I also bite his neck or shoulder when I climax. He keeps complaining about hurting, and feeling humiliated, but he has let me have my way so far. That stopped when I brought home a small whip the other day. He won't let me use it. I have offered him a compromise, he can hit me as well, but he says I'm nuts and there's no way he's going to allow a whip in our bedroom. I think he's overreacting, what's your opinion?

I think your husband isn't into sadomasochistic sex games at all. When he lets you slap and bite him he is already making a compromise. Your offer to let him hit you as well is obviously not tempting for him at all. So offer your partner a real and fair compromise, allow him to do something that he desires himself.

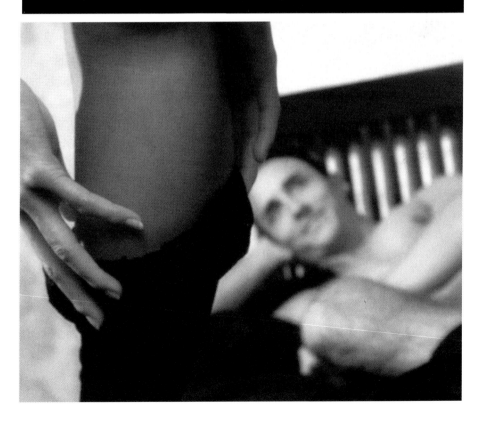

I have fantasised for a while now about being spanked by a woman but I've always been too embarrassed to confide in any woman I have ever been with. Is this a normal fantasy, and would you have any ideas on how I might approach this with a prospective partner, or if I should at all?

One out of every three males has masochistic fantasies. Some like being spanked, others bitten or whipped – there is a wide range of pain inflicting activities that inspire men's (and women's) fantasies. Although your wish isn't that unusual, it wouldn't be wise to mention it on one of the first dates with a new girlfriend, the risk of being dismissed as a 'weirdo' is too big. So wait until you know a woman better, check out her own sexual preferences, then mention your fantasy in a playful way that allows you to pull back in case she's appalled by the idea.

Trying to spice up my marital sex life, I got myself a chastity belt from a sex shop. I couldn't wait to try it out. I spent a romantic evening with my husband, all the time wearing the chastity belt underneath, without him knowing. When he undressed me and found the belt, he got all excited, but his excitement soon turned into impatience and then anger when I told him that I had hidden the key and he needed to find it first. He complained that he didn't have time for silly games, and that he needed to get up early next morning. I was so disappointed. He completely spoilt the game. The key was in my bra, so he would have found it in no time. I feel like giving up on him.

Don't give up yet, talk to your husband about your feelings, I am sure he will apologise for being so impatient. He probably lost his patience when he was sexually aroused, looking forward to making love to you, and then finding out that what he desires is out of reach. Next time, let him know in advance that you are wearing your chastity belt to give him the chance to get into a playful mood and enjoy your game.

25 Sexual Orientation

Our survey revealed that one out of every three Irish women and men have experienced sexual encounters with somebody of their own sex.

Some only kiss and cuddle, others masturbate together or touch each other. More than one out of ten share intimate kisses or have sexual intercourse. Most have their same sex experiences as adolescents, when they are full of curiosity about all sexual matters, and aren't too sure yet what their own preferences are.

Love Between Women

Erotic love between women is one of the mysteries that have kept the fantasies of artists, poets and normal humble souls occupied throughout the centuries. It is hard for many people to imagine what exactly women do with each other when they make love, which intensifies the fascination immensely. Men especially can't understand why women would prefer the company of other females above that of males. Women, however, have a pretty good idea why some women prefer to stick to their own sex. Women see themselves as having more empathy than men. You can talk to women about everything; overall they are more caring and considerate.

For the majority of women, an intimate relationship with another woman might not be their first choice, but it is a lifestyle they might possibly consider for themselves. Less than every second woman (46%) in Ireland can imagine living with another woman as a partner. While only one out of every 25 Irish women regards herself as being homosexual, many more have had sex with a woman. One out of every three has had sexual contacts with another female.

The reasons are manifold, including curiosity, the urge for love and tenderness, being badly disappointed by men, the irresistibility of a female seducer, the desire to try out every possible way to make love, or simply a natural pull towards their own sex.

When women make love to each other, tender caresses and kisses play the main part. Sex toys, like dildos or vibrators, are seldom used. Hands, lips, and tender skin contact are the main sources of pleasure given and received.

A woman's kiss is more tender, more caressing, and less forceful and urgent than a man's. Women can kiss for hours on end, without moving to another stage of their intimacy.

'That is the main difference between kissing a woman and kissing a man,' explains Sylvia (23). 'A man is always hurrying you along, with the hope of getting much more than kisses out of you. It is completely different with a woman. You might end up in bed eventually, but without all the pressure.'

A woman knows how to touch and stimulate another woman. After all, another woman's longings are a mirror of her own. Sometimes, all you want is to cuddle and snuggle up, without having to explain why you are not up to anything more. Another time, you might just want an erotic massage. A female lover doesn't need any explanations – her hands will move expertly over her partner's body, for she knows only too well from her own experience what her lover desires.

The main question people wonder about is how two lesbian women have intercourse, or more bluntly, what can two vaginas do?

There are basically three main ways for women to make love to each other: by touching each other's genitals, by kissing them, or by rubbing them against each other. As you can imagine, there are almost uncountable variations and combinations of lesbian love. One of the most favourite positions is to lie belly to belly, with the legs entangled. You can kiss and caress, look into each other's eyes, while your intimate parts tenderly move against each other. Your hands are free to move all over your partner's body, triggering shivers of pleasure.

Much to the disappointment of the male half of the world, women can well do without penises or their manifold surrogates. Dildos, vibrators and other penis-shaped objects play only a minor part in lesbian lovemaking.

'I often don't understand what these women are up to,' complains Bert (28) from Co. Monaghan. 'They dance with each other in the disco, snog and fumble each other. Have they all turned lesbian all of a sudden, or is that just one of those new tricks girls come up with all the time to confuse us guys?'

Most of the time this is indeed a show to catch men's attention, and it works, doesn't it? Guys are fascinated by lesbian play, and it is one of their dreams to be let in as the third party, so that they can show them what real love is about.

WOMAN TO WOMAN

What women have done with another woman:

Kisses on the mouth	29%
Holding hands	22%
French kisses	19%
Cuddling	14%
Intimate kisses	9%
Necking, caressing of breasts	8%
Petting, caressing of genitals	8%
Sex games with a vibrator	7%
Intercourse	6%

MAN TO MAN

What men have done with another man:

Kisses on the mouth	22%
Masturbating together	20%
French kisses	19%
Holding hands	19%
Petting, caressing of genitals	17%
Intimate kisses	14%
Intercourse	13%
Cuddling	12%
Sex games with a vibrator	11%

Love Between Men

As well as women, many men have sexual experiences with members of their own sex, mainly during adolescence. The range of sexual activities goes from masturbating together, kissing and oral sex to intercourse. Kissing and cuddling plays a slightly lesser role than achieving an orgasm. But then, this difference isn't that huge. It only reflects the different interests that can be observed between so called 'straight' women and men as well.

When people think of gay sex, the first picture that involuntary comes into their mind is often the image of men jumping on each other in a park, or having sex in a gay bar. Sure, there is a small rough scene, but this scene definitely doesn't give a realistic picture of homosexuality. Most homosexual men have completely normal, caring and loving relationships.

In male sexuality, mutual masturbation plays a huge part, as does oral sex. Similar to lesbian couples, they often find their sex life more fulfilling. And again, they have the huge advantage of knowing all about their partner's genitals.

The main difference between gay and lesbian couples' sex lives is that men can have penetrative sex without the use of sex toys. Many homosexual men practice anal intercourse. Some love to receive it; others only like to play the active part, while others don't fancy it at all. Some only play games of anal stimulation without any penetration involved.

Coming Out

Sexual orientation can be confusing and it can be difficult to work out where your sexual preferences lie. It often takes years before a guy or a girl finds the courage to admit to themself that they are homosexual or bisexual. It can take years of wondering, experimenting, and trying to repress their true feelings before they come out. It is so much easier to swim with the main stream.

'At a school reunion, I linked up with an old school friend, who told me she was now sleeping with women. After a few drinks, I told her that my number one fantasy was to be with a girl but that I had never tried it. That night we went home together and had a wonderful time. Since then I feel free to approach other women.' Niamh (28) from Co. Dublin.

Once you are clear about your feelings, and have made the decision to live them out, your next concern is how to tell people. Should you tell your family and friends at all, or just wait until they find out themselves? How will they react? When is the best time to talk to them?

First of all, you don't have to tell anybody, especially if you aren't too clear about your own feelings yet. But if you feel sure, it can be a great relief to tell your trusted best friends, and then your parents as there is a good chance that they will accept and love you the way you are. On the other hand, it's best to be selective about who you tell. The simplest rule is don't tell anybody who you wouldn't usually talk to about other intimate details about yourself.

Be prepared that people might say things that they don't really mean – as a result of not knowing what to say. It might take some of them, especially your parents, a good while to get used to the news.

TIPS

Follow your instincts. If you feel pulled towards somebody of your own sex, give it a chance.

Sex Dictionary

BISEXUAL
Being sexually attracted to both women and men.

COMING OUT
The process of acknowledging and letting others know that you are homosexual or bisexual.

GAY
Another word for homosexual.

HETEROSEXUAL
Being sexually attracted to the opposite sex only.

HOMOSEXUAL
Being sexually attracted only to your own gender.

LESBIAN
Homosexual woman.

STRAIGHT
Another word for being heterosexual.

Q&A

I am confused about my sexual orientation, not knowing whether it's girls or guys I want to be with – how can I tell whether I am straight or gay?

If you feel attracted to both men and women, it might be a good idea to experiment in order to find out whom you want to be with in the long run – it might be men only, women only, or both. One out of every three young men feels sexually attracted to another man at some stage. While most of them stick to being straight afterwards, one out of every ten men remains strongly attracted to guys. About half this group fancy men only and therefore are homosexual, and the other half are bisexual: fancying women and men. You can see that the dilemma you find yourself in isn't unusual at all. Instead of 'sorting your head out', keep an open mind and allow yourself some time to have different experiences.

I am very tempted to try sex with another woman. Should I go for it?

Many women fantasise about making love to another woman, while only about one out of ten fulfil their fantasy. One of the main reasons why women dream about another female is the hope that sex would be less rough and technical, but more tender and loving instead. If you are unattached at the moment and feel tempted to try out lesbian sex, I can't see why you shouldn't go for it. If you are in a relationship, I think it's not fair on your partner to sleep with somebody else, regardless of whether it's a man or a woman.

I caught my husband with another man. Has he become gay all of a sudden?

I very much doubt that your man has become gay all of a sudden, he has probably been attracted to men for a good while, but either suppressed his feelings or wasn't even consciously aware of them. You need to talk to your husband about his feelings to find out whether he is gay or bisexual. If he is bisexual, try to treat his cheating the same way as you would treat a fling with another woman.

I find it more and more difficult to enjoy my husband's lovemaking. I would rather be in the arms of another woman. It is only recently that I've started to have these fantasies. Do you think I'm a lesbian?

I think you are not satisfied with your marital sex life, so you are unconsciously looking for an alternative. When you ask women why they dream of having sex with another woman, the answer you hear most often is the hope that sex would be less rough, more tender and loving. Think about your own reasons for dreaming of other women, and about what you miss or dislike in your marital sex life. Before you go for any sexual experiments, you should try to find out what you're lacking with your partner first to give your marriage another chance.

My boyfriend likes to have a finger up his bum when we make love. Does he have a gay streak, or do straight men like this as well?

Many men like anal stimulation, regardless of their sexual orientation. The anus is a very sensitive area, and many men, both heterosexual and homosexual, love to be touched and teased there. Some just like external teasing, while others fancy anal penetration as well.

I am a completely normal teenager. But I find myself attracted to both lads and girls. I keep my 'gay' side to myself. I just want to know which is the right path to follow? Should I just go with girls or concentrate on guys?

Many teens, especially guys are confused about their sexual orientation, and many try out gay sex. Most end up in heterosexual relationships in the end, only about five per cent stick to being gay, and another five per cent go on loving both men and women. The main reasons for going 'straight' in the end are the wish to have your own family and the pressure of society. This last point isn't much of an issue anymore. Being gay is widely regarded as completely natural and normal, as you will see more clearly as you get older. There is no need to make up your mind now as to what way of life to choose. It's best to follow your feelings until you see more clearly where you stand.

I have been with my girlfriend for three years now. A few months ago I met this gay guy at a party. I felt sexually attracted to him from the first moment I saw him, and he fancies me too. This has never happened to me before – I always thought I was straight. Now I want to sleep with this man, but I don't want to loose my girlfriend either. How can I arrange to have and keep both of them?

If you feel attracted to this man so much, sleep with him and see how you feel about things afterwards. Then you have to make up your mind. In the long run, you can't keep your girlfriend and sleep with a man as well. Your girlfriend wouldn't tolerate that, and it would be unfair to do it behind her back.

At the age of almost 50, I have become extremely attracted to the same sex. I'm divorced with grown up children. I don't feel anything for men anymore; women now are all I want to be with. Is it only a crisis I'm going through, or is it possible that I am lesbian, although I was married for over 20 years? Should I give in to my feelings, as I really want to be with another woman? On the other hand, I'm terrified of how my children and friends might react.

You are an independent woman, so I can't see any harm in doing what you feel like. It is quite possible that you are indeed lesbian;

you wouldn't be the first woman who managed to hide her real feelings and preferences from herself for many years. Even nowadays, homosexual women and men often pretend to be 'straight', giving in to the pressure of family and society, although homosexuality is widely recognised as normal. If you are worried about your family's reaction, don't go public with your feelings before you are really sure about them.

My best mate has told me that he's gay. I was so shocked; he never showed any signs of being homosexual. I told him I don't mind, and promised not to tell anyone. We talked about when he first realised that he was gay, and he said it was when he was 15. And then he confessed that his sexual fantasies are mainly about me. I'm not gay, and have never looked at a man that way. But when my mate told me that he masturbates regularly about me, it really turned me on, and that's my problem. For the past two weeks I couldn't stop thinking about what he said. I know I'm not gay, so why have I become curious, and why am I thinking about having sex with him? Should I try it with him once, as he wants it very much?

Don't rush things. As you said yourself, you have been pretty rattled by your best friend's revelation, so give yourself time to let your tumultuous feelings settle down. Then try to work out why you are tempted to sleep with your best mate. Is it love? Is it sexual curiosity? Or is it a mixture of both? Talk to him about your feelings; be as honest with him as he has been with you. If you want to sleep with him, go for it, but do it for yourself, and not only to please your mate.

26 Keep it Safe

It is so much fun to have sex, and such a nuisance to have to think about birth control and sexually transmitted diseases (STDs) every time our hormone levels hit the roof.

The best thing we can do is to get contraception organised, so we don't have to panic every time we want to make love.

Men don't have much of a choice when it comes to taking responsibility for contraception. It's either using condoms, or having a vasectomy to become sterile. For women the choice is more difficult. To find the right method, it is important to get as much information as possible. Of course the method has to be safe. Ideally, it should be easily available and practical as well.

First of all, it is important to know the possible alternatives. The following shows a short overview of the main methods of birth control that are available.

Hormonal

The Pill

The pill contains two hormones that stop a woman from ovulating. It has to be taken daily, normally with a pill-free break of seven days per cycle. The pill is extremely safe when taken properly. If you take a pill late (more than 12 hours) or even forget it completely, it is not effective anymore. The same can happen if you suffer diarrhoea or vomiting.

Mini Pill

The mini pill contains a hormone that has to be taken exactly at the same time every day. It is almost as effective as the 'normal' pill, but has to be taken by the clock. Delays of more than three hours – as well as diarrhoea or vomiting – make it ineffective.

Chemical

Spermicides

There is a wide range of chemical creams, foams and jellies that are applied into the vagina before inter-course to kill sperm. These chemicals are not very reliable, so they should be used in combination with condoms or other methods. They can also irritate the vagina, causing a burning or itchy feeling.

Barrier

Male Condom

A condom is a sheath of latex that has to be pulled over the penis before intercourse. First time users should practise with a spare condom before they first use it with a partner. To put it on: hold the small reservoir at the top of it between thumb and forefinger, and then carefully unroll the condom over the erect penis. After intercourse, hold the condom in place when you pull the penis out of the vagina. Condoms protect against pregnancy and STDs. In the 1950s the first lubricated condoms were launched. Since then condoms have become thinner and therefore much more comfortable. Another important improvement was made when the manufacturers recognised that one condom size does not fit all. So condoms are now available in different sizes, length and width to fit each individual perfectly. The main problem with the reliability of condoms is the factor of 'human error'. So apply and remove them carefully, and make sure that they aren't out of date. To make condoms safer, you can combine them with a spermicide.

If you use condoms in combination with a lubricant, choose a water-based lubricant that is recommended for condoms. Oil-based lubricants like body lotion or Vaseline can ruin a condom, making it useless. You should always use a condom when you have sex with a new partner.

Female Condom

A female condom, often called 'Femidom', is a strong, but thin condom that you insert into the vagina before intercourse. It has rings on both ends. While you push the ring on the closed side into the vagina, the ring on the open side stays outside.

Diaphragm

A diaphragm is a rubber cap that is placed into the vagina before intercourse to cover the cervix. It has to be used in combination with spermicides to work properly. It is a bit awkward to apply and has to be left in for several hours after sex.

Intrauterine

IUD

An IUD is a tiny intrauterine device that is placed into the uterus by a doctor to stop sperm meeting an egg and to keep fertilized eggs from settling in. IUDs can be kept in place for several years, and are almost as effective as the pill.

Operative

Sterilisation

This method, available for men and women, permanently stops fertility. It is used mainly if couples already have children and don't want any more.

Natural

Coitus Interruptus

The penis is withdrawn from the vagina before the male ejaculates. Semen frequently escapes prior to ejaculation, which makes this method unreliable. In addition, it is highly unsatisfactory for both partners. The male has to concentrate on withdrawing before he comes, while the female worries whether he will make it in time.

Postcoital Shower

Showering directly after intercourse to wash sperm out doesn't do much good. Sperm is much too quick for that. Even if you jump out of bed immediately, some sperm will be well beyond your reach by the time you make it to the shower. This method is extremely unreliable.

Calendar Method (Knaus-Ogino)

To make this method work at least half way, a woman has to record her

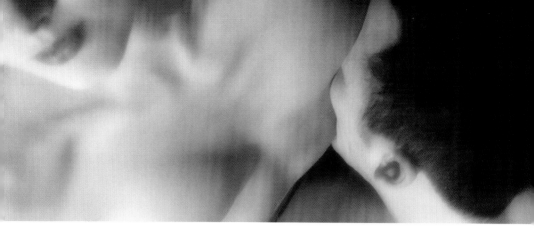

menstrual cycle in a calendar for the period of a year. Based on that, the probable time of the next ovulation is calculated. During the time of a possible ovulation (normally at least ten days), the couple has to restrain from unprotected sex. As a woman's ovulation can change at any time this method is unreliable.

Condoms

Condoms have a long history. Their use can be traced back more than 3000 years, when the ancient Egyptians used a linen sheath as protection against diseases.

The earliest evidence of the use of a condom in Europe dates back almost 2000 years, to the cave paintings of Combarelles in France. The ancient Romans also used condoms. Then there is a huge gap in history. The first written evidence of condoms dates back to the 1500s, when Gabrielle Fallopius (yes, the same man the fallopian tubes were named after) describes a sheath of linen that he has invented to protect men against syphilis. It was only later that their usefulness in the prevention of pregnancies entered the picture.

Over the intervening years condoms became more comfortable when they were made out of animal intestines. Unfortunately they were so expensive that they were often washed and reused, making them much less reliable

Finally, in the 1800s the manufacture of condoms was revolu-tionised by the discovery of vulcanised rubber by Goodyear (yes, the founder of the tyre company) and Hancock. Now condoms could be mass-produced at low costs.

The early 1900s brought the latex condom and with it, a huge increase in sales.

So we have come a long way from the linen sheaths which the history of condoms started with, 3000 years ago. And after 3000 years, you can even legally buy condoms in Ireland.

Sex Dictionary

CONDOM
A sheath of latex that has to be pulled over the penis before intercourse to protect from pregnancy and STDs.

PRE-CUM
Pre-ejaculatory fluid that leaks out of the penis before ejaculation. It can contain a high concentration of sperm.

SPERMICIDE
A sperm-killing substance, mainly used with condoms or in combination with other methods of contraception.

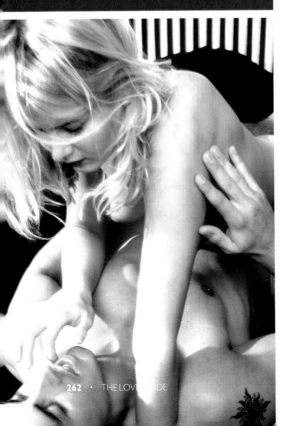

Safer Sex

In the era of AIDS and many other STDs (Sexually Transmitted Diseases), it is vital to protect yourself from infection. Safer sex — not including sexual abstinence — is the best protection. That means: stick to sexual practices that involve a lesser risk of infection with AIDS and STDs. Masturbation and petting would be comparatively safe. Contact with the partner's blood, semen, or vaginal fluids should be avoided, especially if you have a new partner, and don't know anything about their medical background. And of course, always use condoms, either male or female ones. Avoid one-night stands, especially when you have had a few drinks and are not in full control of your, or the other person's actions. This sounds like a horror scenario, but you need to be aware of the risks of having sex without protection.

Q&A

What is the best method of birth control?

Condoms are the only method of birth control that protect not only against pregnancy, but against infections as well. This makes them highly recommendable for men and women who don't have a steady, long-term relationship. Couples who live in a monogamous relationship, and are therefore not at a high risk of catching infections from each other, mainly vote for the pill. The pill is the safest method of birth control, as long as it's being taken regularly, and you don't suffer from vomiting or diarrhoea. Almost as safe, but not as common, are IUDs. These are tiny intrauterine devices that are placed in the uterus by a doctor to avoid pregnancy.

When I really want to have sex, but don't have anything at hand to take precautions: what is the best thing to do? Coitus interruptus?

Don't rely on unreliable methods of birth control that could get you into trouble. Instead, satisfy each other with your hands and lips. If you do it right, mutual masturbation and oral sex are as satisfying as intercourse.

Where can I find condoms that fit?

It is quite easy nowadays to find special sized condoms. The easiest way is to order them over the Internet. If you open a search engine like Yahoo or Google, and search the net for 'condoms to fit', you will find what you are looking for — extra small ones, large fits, slim ones, and many more. You can even get fancy stuff like flavoured condoms, coloured ones and ones that glow in the dark, and so on.

Is it safe to have sex without a condom?

Condoms protect against pregnancy and infections, especially STDs and AIDS. Making love without a condom is only safe if both you and your partner are healthy and live in a strictly monogamous relationship, that means if you both never have sex with other people.

How safe is coitus interruptus?

The withdrawal method isn't safe at all. The failure rate is around 20 per cent per year. That means that out of a 100 women who depend on withdrawal as their only means of birth control, about 20 become pregnant within a year. This method is unreliable because semen often leaks out before a man ejaculates. Coitus interruptus also spoils the fun for both partners. The male has to concentrate and pull back when he's ready to come, spoiling his climax, while the female is worried whether he'll make it in time.

When is it necessary to practise safe sex?

You should always practise safer sex when you can't be absolutely sure that both you and your partner are healthy. Otherwise you are at risk of catching infections, especially STDs that can be life threatening in the worst scenario. A condom is the best way to protect against infections, so the first rule of safe sex is to always use a condom. Also avoid contact with the partner's blood, vaginal fluids, or semen when you sleep with a new person.

What exactly is a Femidom, and how is it used?

A Femidom is a female condom. It is a strong thin condom that has to be inserted into a woman's vagina before intercourse. It has rings on both ends. While you push the ring that's located on the closed side into the vagina, the ring on the open end stays outside. Femidoms are a bit more awkward to handle than male condoms, but with a bit of practise you can get used to them.

Can I get pregnant when I have my period?

Although it is the safest time, it is still possible to become pregnant during your period. So you need protection all the time to be on the safe side.

Can I still get pregnant once my menopause has started or can I stop worrying?

At the beginning of your menopause you can still get pregnant. But if you haven't had your period for a whole year, you can stop worrying about birth control. To make absolutely sure that you aren't fertile anymore, check with your gynaecologist before you take any risks.

For medical reasons, I can't take the pill, so my husband and I need to find another way to prevent pregnancy. As we both like anal sex, the idea was to only have anal sex to make sure I won't get pregnant. But is it safe enough? Or can I get pregnant from anal sex as well?

You can't get pregnant from sperm that is deposited into your anus. There is a very slim chance that leaked out sperm could end up in your vagina, being placed there by fingers, penis or sex toys, but it won't travel there on its own.

Can I get pregnant when we make love in the water, or will the sperm be washed out automatically? It would be very awkward to use a condom, so I'd rather go on the pill if that is necessary.

You can get pregnant when you have unprotected sex in the water, so you'll need to use contraception. You are right, to use a condom would be pretty awkward. If you plan to go on the pill, please consult your gynaecologist for a checkup, and to find the best pill for you.

My girlfriend and I always use condoms when we sleep together, but we first make love without them to feel each other skin on skin, and then put the condom on only shortly before I come. I have noticed that even long before I ejaculate some fluid is leaking out of my penis. Could this make my girlfriend pregnant?

The fluid that is emitted from your penis when you are sexually aroused can contain a high concentration of sperm. This so called pre-ejaculatory fluid, or, in short 'pre-cum', can make a woman pregnant, so it is important that you put on a condom from the very start.

27 Sexual Problems — HER

Most women have concerns about their body, their sexual ability or their inability to achieve an orgasm.

This chapter deals with common female sexual problems and the most frequently asked questions relating to these problems.

Failure to Come

The main sexual problem women suffer from is the failure to achieve an orgasm when they have intercourse. Women naturally take much longer than men to come. One of the reasons is pure anatomy. The penis receives permanent direct stimulation during intercourse, while the clitoris doesn't get much at all. So it is important that a woman is already well aroused, preferably at a level well ahead of her partner, when intercourse starts. Practising cunnilingus is a good way to arouse a woman and allow the man time to cool off.

The best way to make sure you climax is to manually stimulate the clitoris during intercourse. Most women are too shy to do it themselves, others don't even know how to go about it. So first of all, try out on yourself and see which kind of caresses turn you on. Touch yourself experimentally. Then show your man how he can give you a helping hand. Don't expect him to get it right at the beginning. Avoid criticising his efforts, just tell or show him what he could do to increase your pleasure.

'I was almost 30 when I had my first orgasm,' tells Amanda (36) from Co. Dublin. 'I read about how to touch myself in a woman's magazine and it worked. And since I found the courage to show my husband what he can do for me, my sex life has changed from desperate to absolutely perfect.'

Loose Vagina

After childbirth women often complain that their vagina isn't as firm as it used to be. The well known, but simple, Kegel exercises can help you to get back into shape. Contract the muscle in your pelvic floor for a few seconds, then loosen them again, contract them again for a few seconds and so on. Do this two or three times a day and you should feel the results after a few weeks. In case you are not sure which muscle I am talking about: it is the same muscle you use to control your bladder.

Lack of Sexual Interest

Lacking interest in sex is a problem that often starts after childbirth or later on in life with the beginning of menopause. It is often related to hormonal changes, so it is always advisible to consult a doctor about it.

After Childbirth

After childbirth, women often concentrate fully on their new role as a mother, unconsciously neglecting their role as a partner and often their social life as well. One common symptom is neglicence of themselves. To get back on track and back to a normal and satisfying sex life, the first step is to find pleasure again in being a woman, not solely a mother. Look after yourself and take time to care for your partner as well.

Get a babysitter and go out for a night. Don't treat each other as just parents, but as lovers.

Menopause

The change of hormone levels that occur at the onset of menopause can also cause a lack of interest in sex. Another reason for sexual disinterest is that many women feel like they lose their purpose in life when their children are grown up and have left the house or when they retire. They find themselves on their own all of a sudden with a huge vacuum in their life that needs to be filled. This often leads to depression and depression can be accompanied by sexual disinterest.

The best remedy in this case is to remodel your life. Treat yourself to a make over, find new interests, join a club or a group, an evening class, or volunteer for a charity organisation, whatever suits you. Make new friends and try to revive your partnership. Once you are well and happy again, your sexual interest will return as well.

If your lack of interest is caused by your partner, the best thing to do is to encourage him to get into shape as well, if this is what needs to be done.

Another scenario is that your partner has lost interest in you. In that case, think about what might be wrong with your relationship, try to improve what you can do from your side, and if that doesn't help talk to your partner. Avoid criticising or accusing him, that would only push him into a defensive position which wouldn't help your cause.

Dryness

The main reason for vaginal dryness is an insufficient level of sexual arousal. Men can be ready for intercourse within a minute or two, while women need at least 20 minutes until their vagina is sufficiently lubricated. To be on the safe side, allow for at least half an hour of foreplay. Make sure that this foreplay doesn't only consist of her spoiling him, but that he looks after her as well.

Before you move on to intercourse, simply check with a finger whether the vagina is moist enough. If not, stay with foreplay for a while longer. Intimate kisses can help, as well as a direct massage of the clitoris.

If nothing works or you are in a hurry or up for a quicky, use a lubricant.

'We love to have a quicky now and then,' tells Gabriel (29) from Co. Wicklow, 'but my partner doesn't get moist that fast. When we try anyway, it feels like I'm hitting against a brick wall. She now uses lubricant and that always works. Our quickies feel so much better now since I don't have to batter my way in anymore.'

Vaginal dryness is also one of the typical symptoms during menopause. If this problem effects you, discuss it with your gynaecologist.

Other Sexual Problems

Another worry many women share is that their genitals aren't pretty enough. The complaints range from a too small clitoris to big labia and dense pubic hair.

Clitorises as well as labia naturally vary in size but I have seldom heard a man complain about these parts of his girl's anatomy. The only complaints I hear now and then concern a woman's pubic hair. If it is very dense, coarse and long, it can cause discomfort and pain during oral sex and intercourse. But there is an easy way to solve that problem: get a lady shave to trim your pubic hair down to a neat length, and shave off everything that would stick out of a bikini. If you don't like the thought of shaving go to a beautician and get a bikini line wax.

Women also worry about their breasts. Many worry that their breasts are too small and some even consider getting breast implants. They think this will please their man, even if their partner assures them that everything is fine. There are some important factors to consider before you go for transplants. The first is that you need to be fully grown. The next is the fact that implants don't look and feel like real breasts. And of course as in every type of surgery there is a risk involved that things might go wrong. And the last point is that you should never do something as serious as getting breast implants just to please your partner. If you decide to go for it, do it for yourself.

SEX DICTIONARY

KEGEL EXERCISES
Exercises designed to increase the strength of the pelvic muscle. Helpful in cases of vaginal looseness and urinary incontinence.

MENOPAUSE
The time in life when a woman's menstrual cycle ends.

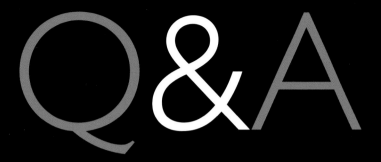

Can clitorises vary in size?

Clitorises can differ in size, the same as penises. The differences aren't as obvious for the simple reason that a clitoris is much smaller to start with. So we aren't talking about differences in the scale of several inches, but only parts of an inch. Another difference in appearance is the way a clitoris is hidden under a hood of skin, not that dissimilar to a man's foreskin.

After giving birth, my vagina isn't as tight as it used to be. Can exercises help to make it tight again?

You can train the muscle inside your vagina with simple exercises, like alternately tightening the muscles for a few seconds, than releasing, then tightening them again and so on. Do this twice per day for five minutes, and it should start to show results after a few weeks. If those exercises don't agree with you, try horse-riding or cycling to tighten your pelvic floor muscles. Strong vaginal muscles not only make you feel tighter, but also allow you to give your partner intimate squeezes when you make love. The right position can also help to make you feel tighter: try having intercourse with your legs closed.

My vagina is so dry that my partner has to force himself in. What can we do to make me moist?

There are two main reasons for a dry vagina. Dryness can be caused by the lack of sexual arousal or it can be one of the symptoms women suffer from when they go through menopause. If dryness is caused by menopause, a gynaecologist can help. If it's caused by lack of sexual arousal, you need to allow more time for foreplay. Men can be ready for intercourse within a couple of minutes, while women often take between 20 and 30 minutes to get physically ready for sex. Delay intercourse for as long as possible by spoiling each other with kisses and caresses. When in a hurry for some reason, use a lubricant. Another reason for vaginal dryness could be that you are having problems in your relationship and don't feel like sex. If this is true think about any problems and discuss them with your partner.

I am always itchy after making love. What could be the reason?

If this itchiness occurs every time you've had sex, the reason could be a fungal infection that affects both you and your partner. Consult your gynaecologist to find out what is causing it. Your gynaecolgist will give you a prescription for an antifungal cream and a suppository to be inserted into the vagina. It is not enough that you alone get treatment, your partner needs to get checked out as well, even if he doesn't show any symptoms, otherwise you could keep infecting each other.

My breasts are very small. Should I go for implants to please my man?

You should consider a breast job only if you have thought long and hard about it and consulted an expert. Don't go for implants just to please your guy. Most men prefer the natural look and feel of small breasts to the unnatural appearance and feel of surgically enlarged ones, so you can't even be sure that your partner would be thrilled with the result of your implant surgery. If you wish to enhance your cleavage, get a wonderbra; they look sexy and can really work wonders on small breasts.

My husband doesn't sleep with me anymore. How can I get our sex life back to normal?

There are many possible reasons for your husband's lack of sex drive. It could be a medical problem. Another possibility is the lack of stimuli in your relationship. Check this out first. Show your husband that you desire him. Dress up sexy and try to seduce him with all your tricks. If that doesn't work, let him know that you aren't happy with your current sex life. Ask him what's wrong with him. If you don't get a satisfying answer, try to get him to see a doctor.

Is it sluttish to shave your pubic hair?

If you shave your pubic hair that doesn't mean you're a slut. If you go to a nudist beach or visit a sauna, you can see that many women trim, style or completely shave off their pubic hair. If you feel uncomfortable about shaving it off completely, go for a bikini trim in front, and only shave the area between your legs. You will see that sex is much more fun that way, with no bristle hair getting in the way. It's completely harmless and has no sluttish element at all.

When I sleep with my boyfriend, it takes at least 20 minutes of foreplay until I get moist enough for intercourse. We both get impatient after a few minutes, and then he has to force himself in, leaving us sore. How can we speed it up?

It is normal for a woman to need 20 minutes to get moist enough for intercourse. If you don't want to wait that long, you or your boyfriend can stimulate your clitoris to speed things up. Or simply apply a lubricant. If you use condoms, it's important to choose a water-based lubricant, others ruin the condom, making it useless.

When I have intercourse I break wind through my vaginal passage. What is causing these half-embarrassing, half-funny noises? Do other women experience them as well?

Other women experience the same thing. It happens when your partner penetrates you fully, and then withdraws completely. This traps air inside you that naturally finds its way out. Don't let yourself be put off by this noise when you make love. If you think about it, there are lots of potentially funny noises involved in lovemaking. If we tried to avoid all those, there wouldn't be much fun left.

Is it true that a woman's vagina elongates to fit the penis in when you have intercourse?

Yes, the vagina not only expands in diameter, it elongates as well when you are sexually aroused. Otherwise we wouldn't be able to enjoy making love, as on average a vagina is shorter than an erect penis.

Is it okay to have sex during my period or do we need to abstain during that time?

If neither of you feels uncomfortable about making love during your period, I can't see a reason why you shouldn't do it. For hygienic reasons, it's better to use a condom when you have intercourse, especially while you are bleeding heavily.

Can my gynaecologist tell when I am sexually excited? Or does arousal only show in a man?

There are visible signs of sexual arousal in a woman that not only gynaecologists can interpret, like a swelling and darkening of the genitals or an increased level of moistness. Don't worry, these symptoms are not as obvious and fool proof as a man's erection.

I can climax when I touch myself, but I can't come when my partner masturbates me, however hard he tries to make me come.

Show your partner how you like being touched. If you know how to make yourself come, you can show your partner as well. To make it easier for yourself to let go and climax at the crucial moment, touch your partner simultaneously.

I have lost all interest in sex. I still love my husband, but don't care about sex anymore. What can I do to get back to normal?

You have taken the first and most important step already, and that is realising that something is wrong and wishing to set it right. To get back to a normal sex life, first think about what you are missing and then talk to your husband about all that you miss and wish for. With a bit of luck, he will be as eager as you to get your love life back on track.

If a man says you are frigid, what does that mean?

If a man says you are frigid, he normally means that you are cold and unfeeling towards him or unable to climax when you sleep with him.

Can the pill make my breasts bigger?

When you begin taking the pill, a swelling of your breasts is one of the possible side effects. Another one is a slight weight gain. These effects should disappear once your body has adjusted to the new hormone level. If they persist, it's normally a sign that your level of oestrogen is too high, which can cause short and long term problems. So you shouldn't take the pill as a method of breast enlargement.

Although I have been married for three years, I have never ever had an orgasm. At first, my husband really tried hard to make me come. Now he has given up and my sex life is becoming more and more frustrating. It can't go on like this, but I really don't know what to do.

First of all try to achieve an orgasm on your own. Most women find it much easier to climax when they masturbate. Once you manage that, you can show your husband how you like being touched. When you make love, choose a position that allows your husband to give you a 'helping hand'.

28 Sexual Problems – HIM

Most men are concerned about their sexual prowess, the size of their penis or how long they can sustain an erection.

This chapter deals with common male sexual problems and the issues men worry about most.

Penis Size

One of men's main worries is that their penis might be too short. Even guys who are medium sized or even above average experiment with useless and potentially dangerous methods of penis enlargement, like stretching, penis weight lifting and using penis pumps. Some methods seem to show a temporary change, but there are none that lead to any long-term improvement. And most are potentially dangerous, as they can cause permanent damage to tissue and blood vessels, leading to impotence in the worst case scenario.

Too Short

The average penis is between six and seven inches long when fully erect, but of course there are deviations in both directions. If you measure at least four inches, there is no need to worry. You can make love in any position you fancy. If you are shorter, there are many positions that allow deep penetration, and make it easy for you to prevent your penis from slipping out. One of the best techniques for short penises is sex from behind, with the woman kneeling in front of her guy. You can hold her hips while you make love to make sure that your penis stays in place.

'My husband's penis measures three and a half inches when erect,' explains Eileen (25) from Co. Dublin. 'The best position for us is doggy style. He never fails to make me come that way. My second favourite is having him lie on his back with his knees pulled up almost to his chin, and then I sit on top of him.'

Too Long

While Irish men mainly worry about their penis being too short, women are more concerned about members that are too big for comfort. It can seriously spoil the fun if he gets in so deep that it causes discomfort or even pain.

The best thing a woman can do to keep a long penis from getting in too deep is to encircle the penis shaft with her hand while making love. Or make love sitting on top of him to take charge. There are also many positions that don't allow a guy to get in all the way. Try to make love with your legs closed or even your ankles crossed. Or lie on your belly or side with him lying behind you.

'My girlfriend loves to look at my big penis, but when it comes to making love it is too big for her taste. We always need to use lots of lubricant, and I have to be careful not to get in too deep. It works best for both of us when she encircles my penis with her hand to control how deep she wants me in,' reveals Eric (36) from Co. Mayo.

Penis Shape

Many men are worried when their erect penis doesn't come up straight, but is bent. A slight bend is not unusual at all, and it is unlikely to cause any problems during intercourse. If the penis is bent so much that it's causing trouble, a small operation can help.

Another frequent worry is the angle of erection. As long as the penis gets erect at all, it doesn't matter much which angle it achieves. Some penises more or less poke out straight when erect, while others lean against the belly. Both variations and everything in between are absolutely normal. Long penises can even point downwards when they are erect.

Premature Ejaculation

Premature ejaculation is a sexual problem mainly young and inexperienced guys suffer from. It basically means that they come too quickly. Some ejaculate more or less on impact, causing a good bit of disappointment and embarrassment. Inexperience and over excitement are the main reasons for premature ejaculation. As it can take a few years for this problem to naturally disappear on its own, here are a few tips which can help a man to last longer.

Ways to Prolong an Erection

1 The easiest way to make you last longer is to masturbate shortly before you have intercourse. On average, the second act takes a few minutes longer. If you come too quickly again anyway, don't turn around and go to sleep, but spoil your girl with your hands and lips until you are ready for another round.

2 Take exercises to gain better control over your body. Masturbate until you are about to come then stop. When your arousal has declined, masturbate again, going a bit further this time, but stop again well before ejaculation. Repeat this five or six times before you finally climax. This exercise will help you to recognise your 'point of no return', the point when it's too late to stop anymore. Once you have control over your 'point of no return', you can take a break during intercourse when you feel it's near and then stimulate your girl in other ways until you have cooled down enough to continue.

3 *The best thing a woman can do in this situation is to encourage her partner to keep caressing her and after a while try to make him erect again. Never criticise him or joke about it while you are in bed together. If it is a real problem and you can't get sexual satisfaction the way things are, talk to your partner about it when you are not in bed. Work out plans that you can try out together. Make him come during foreplay to ensure that he lasts longer during intercourse.*

Tight Foreskin

On a man's erect penis the foreskin should come back all the way over the penis head. If it doesn't this can cause severe discomfort or even pain during intercourse, as the movements of the penis in the vagina pull the foreskin back and forth.

If your foreskin is too tight, don't pull it back by force. Go to an urologist or andrologist to discuss what can be done. If it's not too bad, creams and stretching might solve the problem. In other cases the foreskin can be widened with minor surgery. In severe cases, it can be partly or completely removed (circumcision).

'I suffered from a foreskin that was too tight for more than five years before I finally plucked up the courage to ask my doctor about it,' says William (29) from Co. Tipperary. 'I could masturbate when I was careful, but every time I tried to have sex with a woman, it was a disaster. Especially when I tried to get my penis in – it hurt so much that I couldn't go on. Now everything is great and I enjoy my love life.'

Impotence

Impotence can happen due to several reasons – basically medical or phsychological ones. In young men the failure to gain and maintain an erection is often caused by inexperience, the nervousness of being with a new partner, especially the fear of failing a woman's expectations, and all kinds of stress. Alcohol abuse is a major factor as well. A pint or two can improve your potency because it reduces your worries and makes you more relaxed, but every drink after that can lead to potency problems. Alcohol abuse over many years can even lead to a permanent loss of potency.

In older men impotence is often either caused by a medical reason like diabetes or by the side effects of medication. Of course alcohol, especially the long term effects of alcohol abuse, play a significant role as well.

If you feel that your potency is failing don't hesitate to go to your GP, regardless of your age. Don't take failing potency as a normal sign for getting on in age, as there is almost always a medical or psychological reason behind it and therefore the chance of a cure or at least improvement.

'I thought it was normal for my potency to fail when I was over 60,' explains Martin (64) from Co. Longford. 'It was my wife who urged me to go to my doctor. In the end we found out that a medication he had given me was causing the problem. So we changed the medication, and I was back to a normal sex life within a couple of weeks. And I had given up already, thinking it was old age.'

Strong Sex Drive

Men, on average, have a much stronger sex drive than women, especially when they are under 25. This can lead to many problems in a relationship. The most obvious one is that she feels that he is asking too much of her, especially if he wants sex more often than once a day,

which is not unusual at all. There is even more trouble when she finds out that he is masturbating on the sly, even though they have a regular sex life. Is he a sex maniac, or even a pervert?

Then there is the risk that what he doesn't get at home he finds elsewhere – he goes for one-night stands or even keeps a girl for merely a sexual relationship on the side.

So again, to clear all misunderstandings. A young guy has a stronger sex drive. He might need sex more often than once per day and it's not unusual at all that he goes for it twice in a row. It is also absolutely normal if a man keeps masturbating although he is in a steady relationship and has intercourse regularly.

Excessive Masturbation

Some men masturbate excessively, overdoing it and leaving themselves sore and spoiling the sensation of their orgasms. Masturbating several times a day doesn't cause any permanent physical damage. But you are at risk of getting sore, especially if you don't use a lubricant, and the intensity of your orgasm will recede. You will feel less and less of an orgasm when you come. This can cause you to masturbate again and again, making matters worse.

If you masturbate excessively, the best thing to do is stop for a week to get the full sensation back. Then try to slow down to once or twice per day. You will get more satisfaction out of two quality sessions than you would get out of a dozen rushed ones.

Involuntary Erections

Involuntary erections often happen to guys in their teens. This can cause a lot of worry and can get them into embarassing situations. One of the main worries is that they wake up with an erection in the morning. This is abolutely normal. Another worry is involuntary erections that appear when a guy sees an attractive woman or another man. These erections are normal. The best thing to do in such a situation is to turn your eyes off the sexy sight and think about something utterly unpleasant in order to divert your thoughts.

Involuntary Ejaculations

Another common worry for teenage guys is the fact that they have invol-untary ejaculations in their sleep.

These are called 'wet dreams' and are completely normal. These ejaculations are the male body's natural way of getting rid of sperm that has built up in the testicles. Wet dreams disappear when a man masturbates regularly or has intercourse.

Prolonged Erections

A prolonged erection, also known as priapism, is a condition that doesn't happen too often, but that needs immediate medical attention. If you suffer from an erection that stays for hours and that you can't get rid of or that becomes uncomfortable or painful, visit your GP immediately or go to the nearest Emergency Room. Prolonged erections can lead to permanent damage and loss of potency.

Penis Injuries

Penis injuries also need immediate medical attention, especially if they lead to swelling. The penis is boneless, but it can still be fractured. We speak of a penis fracture when the spongy body of the penis is hurt, causing blood to leak out, resulting in swelling and discolouring. The spongy body is vital to achieve an erection, so any injury to it has to be taken very seriously. If a penis fracture is not treated properly it can lead to permanent damage and even result in impotence.

Rashes

There are lots of other penis related problems; rashes, red blotches or other spots are very common. There is no point in guessing what exactly has caused these problems – always visit your doctor. Don't wait for it to go away on it's own. Even if it does, that doesn't necessarily mean the infection that's causing the symptoms has gone.

Hair Follicles

Another concern that is often mentioned is the growth of hair follicles, especially at the base of the penis. This is normal. These follicles normally don't break out in coarse, long black pubic hair, but only produce short and fair hair that doesn't look odd and doesn't cause any problems.

Blue Balls

This condition is mainly a problem that occurs for teenagers: a pain in their testicles that appears when they have snuggled and fooled around with their girlfriend for hours on end without finding any sexual relief. This phenomenon, 'blue balls', goes away quickly through masturbation.

Sex Dictionary

CIRCUMCISION
Partial or complete removal of the foreskin.

PRIAPISM
A prolonged erection that happens if blood that has assembled in the penis is unable to flow back. Needs immediate medical attention.

PHIMOSIS
A too tight foreskin. This condition often needs medical attention.

WET DREAMS
Involuntary nocturnal emissions of semen – involuntary ejaculations.

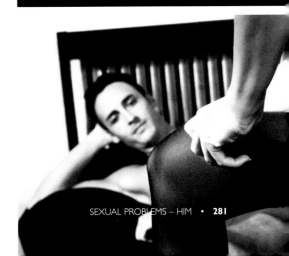

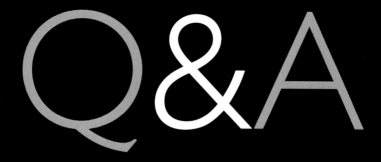

Q&A

My penis is so short that I am afraid to sleep with a woman. What is the average size and how long does my penis need to be to make love?

The average penis measures between six and seven inches when erect. If your penis measures four inches onwards, you are able to make love without hassle. To check your penis size, measure from the bottom of your fully erect penis, from the root up to the very tip. If you fail to satisfy a woman, don't blame the size of your penis, but lack of experience, empathy, and technique. Use your hands and mouth as well as your penis to make your girl come.

Can a penis be too big to fit in?

A penis can be too large, although that doesn't happen often. The vagina is so flexible that it allows even huge penises to fit. To make entrance easier, take your time with foreplay and keep a lubricant at hand. If the penis is so long that it's causing pain by hitting against the cervix, choose a position that doesn't allow full penetration. She can lie on her back, belly or side with her legs stretched out, while he gets in from either front or behind. In other positions, she can encircle the shaft of his penis with her hand to keep him from getting in too deep.

His penis is so small that it keeps slipping out. What's the best technique for short ones?

Try this: when you next make love, pull your knees up and cross your ankles over your man's bum. That way he can penetrate you deeply, and with your legs wrapped around him, you can hold him in position and prevent him from slipping out. If you are athletic, wrap your legs around his neck then hold his bum firmly with both hands to keep him in place.

Is it true that women prefer men with big penises? How long do they want them to be?

Most women prefer average sized penises. When a penis is too big, women are afraid of getting hurt, while when it's extremely tiny, it's less arousing to look at, although it can do as good a job as a big one. So I wouldn't say that size doesn't matter at all, but it's definitely overrated. What matters much more than size is technique.

Is it possible to enlarge my penis naturally, with weight lifting, stretching or other methods?

Weight lifting, stretching or other penis exercises won't make a measurable, permanent difference. As a normal reaction to touching, stroking and squeezing the penis looks bigger while you're exercising, but it shrinks back to its normal size afterwards. These methods are not only ineffective, but potentially dangerous as well as they might cause permanent damage. In the worst scenario this can cause a loss of potency. I am aware of how crucial it seems to be for a guy to be well equipped, but please take my word for it that women find other values much more important.

My erect penis is bent like a banana and looks odd. What can be done?

Most penises don't come up straight when erect, but bend either to the left or right, or even curve inwards towards the belly. As long as it doesn't hinder sexual intercourse there is no reason to do anything about it. When it's causing problems, a small operation can help in most cases. Consult an urologist or andrologist to discuss the details.

My foreskin is so tight that I can't pull it back over the head of my penis. Will I need surgery?

On a fully grown erect penis, the foreskin should come back all the way until the head of your erect penis is fully exposed. If pulling it back is causing discomfort or is even impossible, don't force it back yourself but consult a doctor. A too tight foreskin, also called phimosis, can sometimes be cured by a combination of applying creams and stretching. If that doesn't help, it can often be treated with minor surgery to widen the tight opening. Another solution many men go for is a partial or complete circumcision.

I always come too quickly. What is the best remedy for premature ejaculation?

The easiest way to ensure that you last longer is to masturbate before you have intercourse. Another method is to stop moving before your arousal reaches the so called 'point of no return', when you aren't able to stop yourself from ejaculating. To find your 'point of no return' stimulate yourself until you are close to orgasm, then stop and start again after you have cooled off a bit. Every time you start again, bring yourself a bit closer to orgasm. After a few weeks, you will know exactly at which point you have to stop. Instead of masturbating, you can also practise this technique with your partner.

What are the main factors that cause impotence and what can be done to enhance a man's potency?

Medical as well as psychological reasons can be responsible for failing potency. While in older men medical reasons like diabetes or bad circulation are predominant, it's mainly psychological factors like stress or the fear of failure that cause impotence in younger men. In all age groups, alcohol and drug abuse take their toll. The best way to enhance your potency is a healthy life style. Above all, avoid greasy food, alcohol and cigarettes. If you suffer from impotence, you should consult a doctor for a check up, whatever age you are. Impotence should never be dealt with as inevitable when you are getting on in years. There is almost always another reason behind it.

My penis is covered in itchy red spots. Can I find help without seeing a doctor?

The symptoms you describe could be an allergic reaction, or they could be caused by some STD – there are many possibilities. There is no point in trying to treat this yourself, especially as the wrong treatment could make your symptoms even worse. Go to a doctor to get this checked out. If you are too embarrassed to consult your GP, go to an urologist or andrologist, these are specialists who see symptoms like yours every day. You need to refrain from sexual intercourse until this has been sorted out.

Can Viagra help me to regain my potency? Where can I buy it?

Viagra is a very effective medication that has helped millions of men to regain their potency, and it might be the solution for you as well. To make sure Viagra won't cause you any harm, you need to get a medical check up and your doctor's okay first. If Viagra is suitable for you, your doctor will give you a prescription and you can then buy Viagra at any pharmacy.

When I snuggle with my girlfriend for a few hours, my balls begin to hurt, although she never touches them. Otherwise they are okay. What is wrong, and can I do something about it?

What you describe is a phenomenon called blue balls. It is caused by a congestion of blood in the testicles that occurs when you are sexually excited for a long time without finding any relief. The easiest way to cure this is by masturbating.

I want to sleep with my girlfriend every day, often even twice. Is that okay, or can too much sex be harmful?

You can have sex as often as you wish, as long as it feels good. Making love isn't unhealthy or harmful, on the contrary, it's been proved that men and women who have an active and fulfilling sex life are happier and healthier than those who make love less often. The only potential problem I can see is that a man's sex drive is normally much stronger than a woman's, meaning your lover might not want sex as often as you. If that's the case, make sure to show her that it's not pure sex you're after, but that it's her you long for.

I tried to sleep with my girlfriend for the first time, but was too nervous to get an erection. What can I do to make sure this doesn't happen again?

Many guys fail to get a proper erection when they try to sleep with a girl for the first time. The main reason is inexperience, mixed with nerves and the anxiety about failure. Very often, too much alcohol plays a role as well. While a few drinks might give you courage, they have a damaging effect on your potency. So next time you try, avoid alcohol. Ask yourself whether you really feel ready and comfortable sleeping with your partner. If you do make sure you know how to put on a condom. Explore your girlfriend's body before you sleep with her and become familiar with her anatomy. If you're that well prepared, I am sure you won't have a problem obtaining and sustaining an erection.

I get an erection about 12 times per day, which can get me into embarassing situations. What can I do to control my involuntary erections?

Naturally, the amount of involuntary erections you experience will decrease in time as you get older. To keep you out of embarrassing situations, don't allow yourself to get carried away by erotic thoughts. Force yourself to think about something unpleasant when you feel that an involuntary erection is on its way. This is the best and easist way to prevent them.

Is it normal for a guy to come in his sleep?

For a guy who doesn't have a steady relationship or an active sex life, it is absolutely normal to ejaculate in his sleep at least every few weeks, especially if he doesn't masturbate regularly. If there is no sexual relief of any kind, the body gets rid of the assembled sperm during a nocturnal emission. The best way to avoid these involuntary ejaculations at night is to masturbate now and then to find relief.

I've noticed that there are many hair follicles growing on my scrotum and penis. How do I get rid of them? I am really worried about this, especially as they appear to be multiplying.

It is normal to have hair follicles on the scrotum and the penis, especially near the base of the penis shaft. Don't worry too much as it's unusual for those hair follicles to produce coarse dark hair. It's mostly very fine and tiny hair that grows out of them.

Lately I've got a strong erection out of the blue, without even thinking about sex. When it happened I couldn't get rid of it. It took hours to go away and was very uncomfortable and even painful in the end. What can I do if this happens again?

If this happens again, go to a doctor immediately. What you describe sounds like priapism, which is a prolonged erection that happens if blood has assembled in the penis and is unable to flow back. This can be caused by a medical condition as well as by certain medications. It is a good idea to visit a doctor before it happens again, as this condition can cause permanent damage.

Our national survey revealed many intimate details about Irish people's sex lives. It appears that what was once considered a sexually conservative, almost shy society has now changed. The statistics highlight the fact that many Irish people now have a relaxed, positive and carefree attitude to sex.

In the last few years new sexual trends have emerged and the Irish have welcomed them with great enthusiasm: using sex toys, experimenting with new positions in different locations and talking dirty online are just some of the many things that have spiced up Ireland's sex life. Some people in Ireland are very curious and willing to experiment. Swapping, playing kinky games and one-night stands have become a lot more common and are no longer something that just happens in other countries or in porn films. They have been established in a secure niche of their own.

In general, the Irish have become more comfortable with their sexuality and want to fulfil their sexual wishes, desires and fantasies. The social climate is one of interest, expectation, and open-mindedness towards all sexual matters. But unfortunately, despite changing attitudes in Ireland, people can still find it difficult to reveal their intimate feelings. There is still a great reluctance to talk openly about the joys, problems or anything to do with a couple's sex life. Even among friends, most Irish people clam up and prefer to keep their sexual thoughts, feelings and questions to themselves. There is no need to share every intimate detail about your love life with other people, but it can be very inspiring to talk openly about your special fields of interest, as well as your concerns, to exchange experiences and broaden your horizons.

Most of all it's important to share your intimate thoughts and wishes with your partner. There are still way too many couples in Ireland who sleep beside each other every night without having the faintest idea about each other's sexual longings. Of course before this can be done it is important to immerse yourself in your role as a sexual being. Clarify your own needs and wishes; then think about the best ways to communicate them to your partner. Sharing wishes and fantasies can spice up your sexual relationship and strengthen the emotional bond between you.

Until this level of communication and increased intimacy is achieved one-night stands will continue to increase in popularity. One of the main reasons for this is because it is often easier to open up to a stranger, where there is no emotional attachment, than to a long-term lover. Men and women can then act out their secret dreams, pretend to be somebody else, talk dirty, have kinky sex, share their sexual desires or essentially do whatever they want. While one-night stands can be sexually liberating they can also be dangerous. A major concern is unprotected sex. Young people especially tend to throw caution to the wind, taking risks with unprotected sex that can result in unwanted pregnancies and infection with STDs. The solution is to play it safe – always carry condoms – don't depend on your partner for the night to look after protection and consult a doctor immediately if you develop anything unusual.

As Ireland becomes a more sexually liberated society people's attitudes should continue to change. To help achieve this it is important that whenever you are in trouble, or have a question that intrigues or bothers you, don't be shy about seeking help. There is nothing worse than having to deal with your problems on your own. Confide in your partner, your best friend, your parents, your doctor, your favourite sex agony aunt or any other person you trust to let them help you sort things out.

During my work on this book I have met many Irish people who were reluctant to talk about their sexual interests and problems at first, but who opened up after a while and were brimming over with ideas for topics to discuss. Thanks to everybody who took part, from the first stages of brain-storming and research, to the last stages of discussing the results of our survey. Your contribution of ideas and intimate personal experiences was vital to illus-trate, and give life, to all the statistical figures in this Love Guide.

Dr Angela Brokmann